The Healthy Eating Handbook for Yukon First Nations

by

Vanessa M. Nardelli and Eleanor E. Wein

2nd Edition 1998
Edited by: E.L. Maloney and C.S. Mason

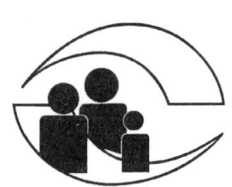 Community Issues in the North

Canadian Circumpolar Institute
University of Alberta
Edmonton, Alberta

About the authors:

Vanessa M. Nardelli has a B.Sc. (Food and Nutrition) from the University of Alberta, and is a member of the Canadian Dietetic Association and the Alberta Registered Dietitians Association. She previously developed a nutrition and diabetes education kit with the First Nations people of Treaty Six, Alberta. Vanessa is currently the Nutrition Educator with the Aboriginal Diabetes Wellness Program in Edmonton.

Eleanor E. Wein has a Ph.D. (Applied Human Nutrition) from the University of Guelph, and is a member of the Canadian Dietetic Association. She has studied food patterns and nutrient intakes of aboriginal people in Alberta, Northwest Territories and Yukon.

About the front cover:

Ram's horn spoon with soapberries and paddle, used to make Indian ice cream. Artifacts kindly supplied by R. Chambers. Photo: E.E. Wein. Background - Blackberries (Mossberries), a traditional source of vitamin C. Photo: R.W. Wein.

Canadian Cataloguing in Publication Data

Nardelli, Vanessa M.
    The Healthy Eating Handbook for Yukon First Nations

ISBN 1-896445-01-2

1. Indians of North America--Yukon Territory--Nutrition. 2. Indians of North America--Yukon Territory--Food. 3. Nutrition --Yukon Territory. I. Wein, Eleanor E. (Eleanor Elizabeth), 1944- II. Canadian Circumpolar Institute. III. Title.

E78.Y8N37 1996   641.1'089'9707191   C96-910269-0

Copyright 1996, 1998 Canadian Circumpolar Institute (CCI) Press
1996 Edition printed by Riley's Reproductions & Printing Ltd, Edmonton AB Canada
1998 Edition printed by Quality Color Press, Edmonton AB Canada

Preface

The overall goal of *The Healthy Eating Handbook for Yukon First Nations* is to encourage development of positive attitudes and skills for healthy eating and balanced lifestyles among Yukon First Nations people. The two main objectives of this work are:

1. To provide information on the nutrient values and benefits of traditional and market foods.

2. To provide nutrition education activities that will help readers develop the knowledge and skills required to choose healthful diets.

The handbook is intended as a resource for Yukon First Nations workers, such as Community Health Representatives (CHRs), Community Health Nurses (CHNs), social workers, teachers, teachers' aides and cultural educators. Information is presented mainly as learning activities that can be adapted for various audiences and age groups. Selected pages are intended as handouts, which may be copied and distributed to group participants.

The idea for this handbook arose from a research project in traditional food use in Yukon. A food and nutrition study was requested by three First Nations, for the purpose of documenting traditional food use as a component of the contemporary diet of Yukon First Nations peoples. Although the illustrations and examples used in this handbook are taken from the communities that took part in this study, the healthy eating concepts can be applied to any community.

Many Yukoners and others contributed to this handbook. They are acknowledged on the following page. We apologize if we have somehow missed naming any of the many contributors.

Acknowledgements

We acknowledge, with appreciation the Yukon First Nations people who contributed their suggestions and ideas during the development of *The Healthy Eating Handbook for Yukon First Nations*, and/or who tested the learning activities designed for this purpose.

The following people deserve special thanks:

Gina Alaric	Denise Marion
Barbara Atkinson	Debbie Mauch
Ken Bear	Isabel McClements
Stella Boss	Edwin McGinty
Glen Bunbury	Eric Morris
Joanne Charlie	Kelly Morris
Carol Christian	Mary Peter
Jim Clark	Gordon Reed
Kathy Edwards	Liz Rowlands
Barb Eikland	Marion Schafer
Rebecca Fenton	Corinne Sheldon
Graham Humphries	Kim Smarch
Betsy Jackson	Roger Smarch
Cheryl Jackson	Alayne Squair
Marvin Johnson	Alena Straka
Kelly Johnston	Mary Rose Sydney
Vicky Josie	Carol Thomas
Minnie Jules	Andrea Underwood
Christine Kuzyk	Maureen Wheelton
Kyle Keenan	Bruce Wiseman

The authors also thank the following nutrition and education professionals who kindly reviewed and commented on earlier drafts of the handbook:

Sharlene Clarke (Dietitian, Whitehorse General Hospital)
Judy Halladay (Nutritionist, Alberta Region)
Sharon Jacobs (First Nations Education Consultant, Whitehorse)
Liz Rowlands (First Nations Health and Social Liaison Worker, Whitehorse General Hospital)

Funding was provided by a Vice-President (Research) Circumpolar Research Grant from the University of Alberta (CCI) to E.E. Wein, and a SEED (Summer Employment/ Experience Development) grant from Employment and Immigration Canada to the Canadian Circumpolar Institute for V.M. Nardelli's summer program. Copy of *Canada's Food Guide to Healthy Eating*, included as Appendix I was kindly provided by Health Canada.

TABLE OF CONTENTS

	Page
PREFACE	i
ACKNOWLEDGEMENTS	ii
TABLE OF CONTENTS	iii
INTRODUCTION	3
Foods from the Past	3
Current Food Patterns	5
Purpose	6
Objectives	6
Teaching Tips	7
FOOD AND NUTRIENTS FOR OUR BODY	9
Food Groups	9
Examples of Traditional and Market Foods	10
Canada's Food Guide to Healthy Eating	11
Recommendations	12
Nutrients for Our Body	13
Macronutrients	13
Micronutrients	13
Other Dietary Components (Dietary Fibre, Water)	14
Nutrients for Special Emphasis	15
Calcium	15
Dietary Fibre	16
Dietary Fat	17
Food Safety	19
SPECIAL DIETARY CONCERNS	21
Heart Disease	22
Diabetes Mellitus	23
Lactose Intolerance	24
SPECIAL NEEDS THROUGH THE LIFE CYCLE	25
Pregnancy	26
Infant Feeding	28
Breastfeeding	28
Formula Feeding	29
Introducing Solid Foods to Infants	31
Elders	32
Nutrition for the Elderly	32
Making Food Easier to Eat	33

	Page
GAMES AND ACTIVITIES	35
Food Group Photo Game	36
Food Group Review	37
Nutrient Bingo	38
Bingo Game Sheet	39
Master Card	40
Cards 1 to 5	41
Fireweed Potato Salad	44
Bingo Handout	45
Calcium Tips	46
Adding Calcium to Our Meal Can be Easy	46
Cooking with Calcium	47
Quick and Easy Casserole	47
My Favourite Salmon Chowder	48
Fibre Everyday!	49
Making Fibre a Part of Every Meal	50
Cooking with Fibre	51
Hearty Carrot Muffins	51
Grandma's Cranberry Muffins	52
Filling Up on Fibre	53
The Fibre Game	55
Fibre Review	56
Cutting Down on Total Fat	57
Total Fat Quiz	59
Fat Review	60
Learning from Elders	61
The Snacking Game	62
Healthy Snacks	63
Community Action	64
Activity Day	64
Community Walk-athon	65
Community Dance-athon	65
Community Clean Up	65
Sofa Aerobics	66
General Evaluation for Games and Activities	67
ADDITIONAL RESOURCES	68
REFERENCES	69
Figure Captions for Back Inside and Outside Cover	70
APPENDIX I: Canada's Food Guide to Healthy Eating	71

INTRODUCTION
Foods from the Past

Years ago Yukon First Nations people consumed only foods harvested directly from the land and water. The availability and abundance of food were not always consistent; therefore, food was shared throughout the community. Fishing, hunting, and gathering methods of the past involved much physical activity and endurance. A great deal of energy was used for these activities, and that, with healthy eating, contributed to a balanced lifestyle. Traditional diets consisted of wild animal, fish, and plant foods that provided essential energy and nutrients for survival. Moose and caribou and, in some areas, sheep, provided most of the meat.

Meat was available throughout the year because preservation methods were adopted that permitted long-term storage. In addition to boiling and roasting, meat was also dried to preserve it for longer periods of time. Dry meat eaten with fat was a popular meal or snack food. Occasionally, the tender meat of an unborn calf was given to the elders as a special treat and symbol of respect (McClellan 1987). Meat, organs, and especially the head or leg bones with marrow, were made into soups or stews. Before the availability of pots and kettles, soups and other foods were cooked in "pots" fashioned from animal skins.

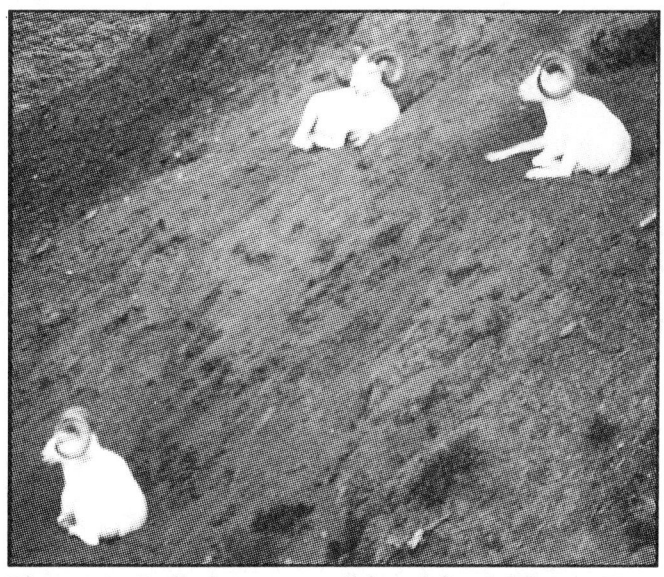

Figure 4. Dall sheep, a traditional food (Photo: R. Chambers).

Smaller animals and birds also contributed to the Yukon diet. Mammals used for food included gophers (Arctic ground squirrels), snowshoe hare, beaver, porcupine, muskrat, mountain sheep and goat. The availability of these animals varied with location, habitat, and season. Birds included ptarmigan, goose, duck, swan, and grouse. Birds provided not only a source of meat, but also eggs.

Another very important food source was fish. Chinook, chum, sockeye, and coho salmon, whitefish, jackfish (northern pike), Arctic grayling, trout, and loche or ling cod (burbot) were species common to Yukon. Usual preparation methods included roasting, frying, and boiling (for fish head soup). Fish was preserved by drying and, in later years, by canning or freezing. An added advantage to the canning process was that it softened fish bones, making them edible - an excellent source of calcium. Fish eggs were considered a delicacy, and were eaten raw, boiled, dried, or fried in fish fat and spread on bannock.

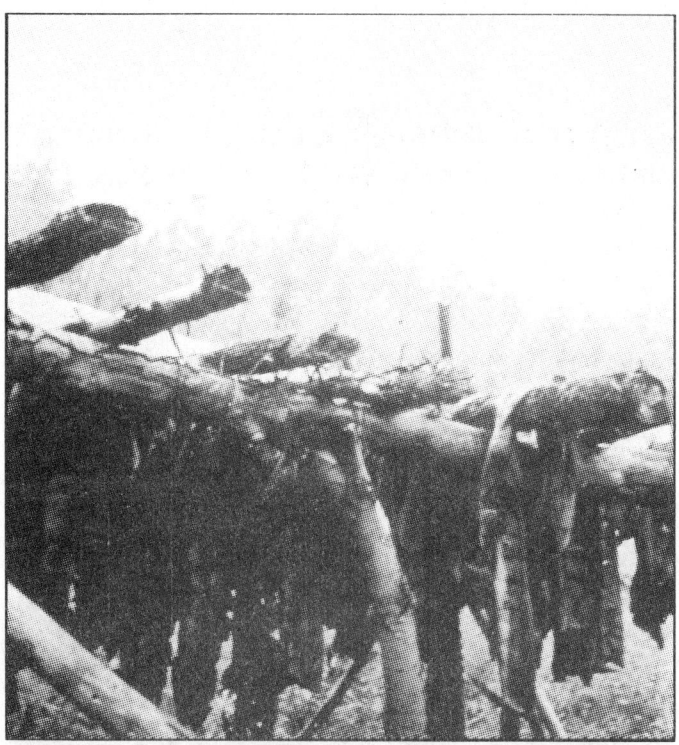

Figure 5. Drying fish - a traditional preservation method still used today (Photo: Department of Fisheries and Oceans.)

Wild plants also constituted an important component of the Yukon First Nations diet. Edible berries included the blackberry, cranberry, blueberry, soapberry, bearberry, rosehip, saskatoon berry, and red currant. Berry picking or "berrying" was an enjoyable task, usually done by women and girls (McClellan 1975). Berries were dried, mixed with fat, and then stored for later use as snacks. Sometimes they were mixed into bannock dough, or made into jams. Other wild plant foods included wild onions, arctic dock, fireweed shoots and leaves, dandelion leaves, wild rhubarb, and bear root. Labrador tea leaves, and the inner bark scrapings and resin or sap of balsam fir and spruce trees were used for nutritional or medicinal purposes.

Although the traditional diet consisted of a variety of foods that supplied most required nutrients, the diet may have been limited in certain nutrients such as calcium and dietary fibre, that are now obtained primarily from market foods. In traditional times, milk was not a staple of the diet, and more or less limited to breastfeeding infants. Older children and adults obtained calcium from other foods, such as fish head soup, or by chewing on the soft spongy ends of moose or caribou bones, and whole fish heads and bones. This was especially important for nursing mothers who required more calcium.

In the past, preservation and preparation of food required much ingenuity. Birchbark baskets or "pots" made of dried caribou stomachs and/or bladders were used as storage containers for berries (McClellan 1987). Berries were mixed with animal grease to retain moisture and nutrients. Fish was cut into small strips and dried on racks over a small fire of cottonwood, which also helped keep the flies away (McClellan 1987). Salmon heads or whole gophers were sometimes stored underground until fermentation occurred, producing a cheese-like substance (McClellan 1975).

Despite the difficulties they faced, earlier generations of Yukon First Nations people met these challenges of providing for themselves and their communities. They survived in large part by consuming traditional foods from many sources in their environment.

Current Food Patterns

Today Yukon First Nations people eat both traditional and market foods. Traditional foods, however, continue to be important, not only from a dietary point-of-view, but also culturally. Moose, caribou, and salmon are still dietary staples (Wein 1994, Wein and Freeman 1995). The amount harvested varies, depending on location. Almost all parts of the animal are eaten, including the heart, kidney, tongue, liver, intestines, bone marrow, head, and nose. Soups, stews, sausages and roasts are common moose and caribou dishes. Ducks, geese, ptarmigan and grouse also contribute occasionally to the modern diet. Berries such as blackberries (mossberries), low and high bush cranberries, blueberries, soapberries, raspberries, and strawberries are also eaten. Labrador tea, balsam fir inner bark tea, and bear root ("Indian sweet potatoes") are still consumed by many people (McClellan 1987). In contrast to long ago, some animals may be less available due to an increased human population and environmental changes such as the installation of highways, mining activities, pollution, and the growth of urban centres such as Whitehorse, having reduced the size of wilderness areas, and therefore hunting grounds.

Market foods can be used to balance a contemporary Yukon First Nations diet. In particular, milk products, whole grain products, fruits, and vegetables provide nutrients which are in limited supply in the traditional foods most commonly eaten today. Milk, cheese, yogurt, and ice cream provide calcium, a nutrient which was probably limited in the traditional diet. These dairy products also provide vitamin A and riboflavin. Milk is an excellent source of vitamin D. Grain products such as whole grain breads, pasta, rice, and cereals provide dietary fibre, thiamin, riboflavin, niacin, and small amounts of iron. Although it does not provide dietary fibre, "enriched" white flour also provides thiamin, riboflavin, niacin, and iron.

The availability of prepared and prepackaged foods such as canned and frozen soups, meats, fish, vegetables, and fruits allows people to stock up on some foods for long periods of time. This is convenient for those who shop infrequently, or live at a distance from a store, since they can eat these foods when traditional foods are in short supply.

Market foods should be chosen wisely. Many are quite high in fat, sugar, and/or salt, and low in fibre (e.g., potato chips, candy bars, carbonated drinks, high fat baked goods such as cakes and doughnuts, fish and chicken deep fried in batter). Eating too many of these foods, in large quantities is unhealthy. Market foods are preserved using methods quite different from those of the past. For example, canned soups, stews, and macaroni are convenient foods to store, and are quickly prepared. Canned and dried soups, however, usually contain large amounts of salt, and therefore should be eaten in moderation. On the other hand, canned fruits, vegetables, and baked beans provide many nutrients and contain little or no added fat. The soft texture of canned fruits and vegetables can be especially good for those who have problems chewing - infants and elders, for example. For infants, soft home cooked vegetables (without added salt), and cooked or canned fruits are best. The amount of salt contained in regular canned vegetables is too high for infants.

Although both traditional and market foods are now available, some Yukon First Nations people are not getting enough of certain vitamins and minerals, while they are getting too much fat in their diet. According to a recent study of three Yukon First Nations in four communities (Wein 1994, 1995, 1996; Wein and Freeman 1995), the present Yukon First Nations diet, on average, meets the health recommendations for protein, vitamins B6, B12, phosphorus, iron, thiamin, riboflavin and niacin. However, it is limited in folate, calcium, vitamins A and D, and in some cases, vitamin C and zinc. More older than younger adults, and more women than men are not getting enough of these nutrients. Furthermore, many people are getting too much fat in their diet. Increasing awareness of healthy eating and balanced lifestyles among Yukon First Nations people of all ages is the first step toward improving nutrition and health.

Purpose

The overall goal of *The Healthy Eating Handbook for Yukon First Nations* is to promote the development of positive attitudes and skills toward healthy eating and balanced lifestyles. One main objective is to provide information on the nutrient value and benefits of traditional and market foods. Another is to offer educational activities that assist in developing skills required to choose healthful diets.

The handbook is intended as a resource for First Nations Community Health Representatives (CHRs), Community Health Nurses (CHNs), social workers, teachers, teachers' aides, and cultural educators involved with health and education programs. Information is presented as group learning activities that can be adapted for various audiences and age groups. Selected handout sheets are intended for photocopying and distribution for group discussion and use.

Objectives

The specific **objectives of the handbook** are:
1. To **promote healthy eating** among Yukon First Nations people by illustrating choices in four food groups that will provide balance and variety in the diet, using traditional and market foods available in Yukon.
2. To provide information to better understand the **special dietary needs** of pregnant and lactating women, infants, and elders.
3. To increase awareness of the risk factors that contribute to **heart disease, diabetes mellitus** and **osteoporosis**, and to provide a means of prevention.
4. To increase awareness of the **role of calcium** and its food sources, and to encourage greater dietary intake of calcium.
5. To increase awareness of the **role of dietary fibre** and its food sources, and to encourage greater dietary intake of fibre.
6. To increase awareness of the **roles of vitamins A, D,** and **folate**, and to encourage greater intakes of these nutrients.
7. To increase awareness of **dietary fat**, and some means of controlling fat intake.

Teaching Tips

As educators, we sometimes forget important tips that can help in teaching; the following **Teaching Tips** may be helpful. "Take home" handout sheets summarize information presented in the sessions.

1. Since communication is a two way process, **educators and participants should have equal opportunity to share thoughts** and be heard. Discussions are usually more open if participants sit in a circle.

2. Appreciate that **participants have at least a basic knowledge** about the topic of discussion. Provide everyone an opportunity to first tell what they already know about the subject of discussion.

3. Respect each **individual's ideas and suggestions**.

4. Encourage **group discussion**.

5. Try to provide the information at a manageable pace, since **knowledge is better retained when studying is approached in small steps**.

6. Encourage the group to **repeat, review,** and **summarize** the information presented at each session.

7. Provide **positive feedback** at all stages of learning.

Starting a group discussion can be difficult, especially if group members have not developed a trust with each other or with the educator. Icebreakers can be useful tools that can enhance the humour, trust, and enjoyment among the group.

Examples of **Icebreakers:**

Encourage everyone to share with the group:

1. one of his/her favourite foods.
2. a particularly memorable feast or celebration.
3. a favourite activity or hobby.
4. his/her expectations of the group sessions.

If participants seem to feel uneasy about taking part in the activities, or Icebreakers, it is best not to force the issue. Maybe share your ideas with them first. Usually, this will bring about discussion in a less threatening way.

FOOD AND NUTRIENTS FOR OUR BODY

The objectives of this section are:

1. To illustrate the **four food groups** with examples of **traditional and market foods**.
2. To recommend ways of providing **variety, balance, and moderation** in the diet.
3. To describe the **nutrients** that our bodies need for energy and health.
4. To describe the role and food sources of **calcium**.
5. To describe the role and food sources of **fibre**.
6. To describe the different types of **fat**.
7. To provide guidance about **food safety**.

Food Groups

What are the four food groups?

1. Grain Products
2. Milk and Calcium Products
3. Vegetables and Fruits
4. Meat and Alternatives

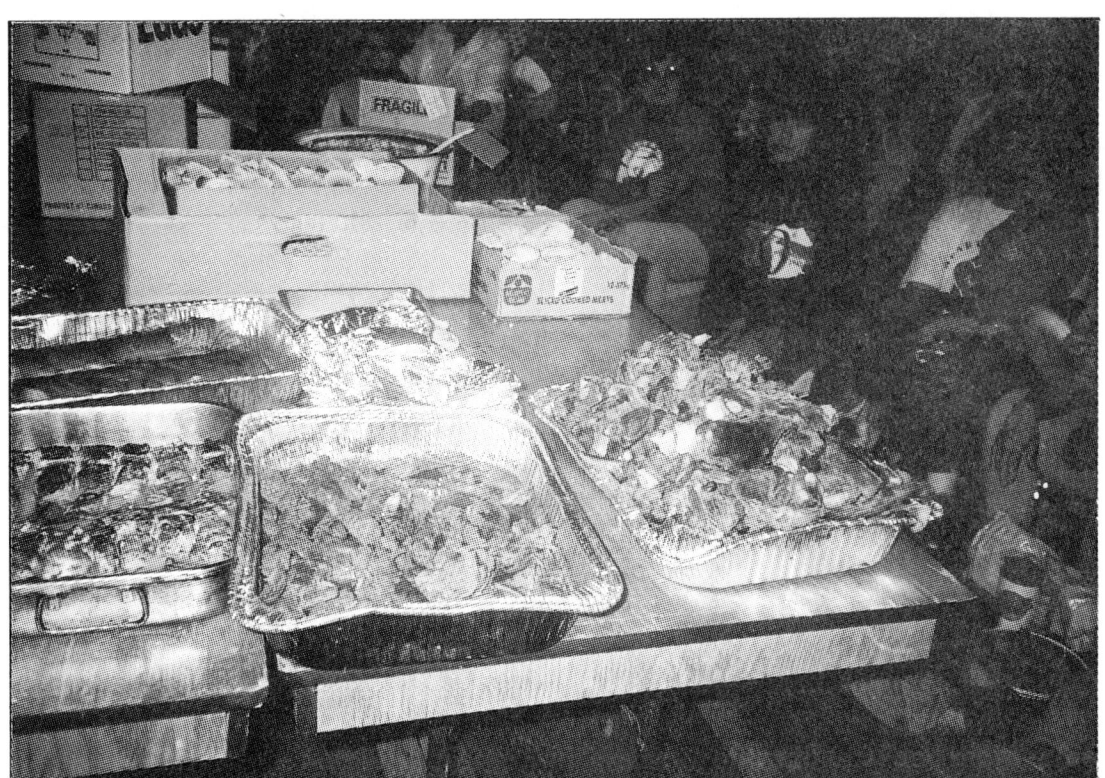

Figure 6. The meat and alternatives group was abundant at this feast in Old Crow. What food groups are missing from this photo? (Photo: V.M. Nardelli).

Examples of Traditional and Market Foods

1. Grain Products

- Bannock
- Wild Rice
- Bread
- Noodles
- Cereals
- Crackers
- Pilot Biscuits
- Oatmeal
- Long or Short Grain Rice

2. Milk and Calcium Products

- Yogurt
- Milk
- Fish Bones
- Cheese
- Fish Head Soup
- Canned Fish with Edible Bones

3. Vegetables and Fruits

- Berries
- Wild Onions
- Apples
- Oranges
- Fireweed Leaves
- Turnip
- Potatoes
- Tomatoes
- Carrots
- Squash
- Lettuce
- Fruit/Vegetable Juice
- Bear Root
- Rhubarb
- Arctic Dock
- Green and Yellow Beans

4. Meat and Alternatives

- Moose
- Baked Beans
- Stews
- Beaver
- Seeds and Nuts
- Gopher
- Geese
- Ptarmigan
- Duck
- Poultry
- Lake Trout
- Ham
- Peanut Butter
- Organs (e.g. tongue, heart, liver)
- Egg
- Moose Sausage
- Caribou
- Split Pea Soup
- Fish Head Soup
- Salmon

5. Other Foods

Note: Many of the following **Other Foods** are high in fat and/or sugar and low in vitamins and minerals. These foods should be avoided or limited in the diet.

- Candy
- Popsicles
- Pop
- French Fries
- Potato Chips
- Chocolate Bars
- Doughnuts
- Coffee
- Cakes

Alcohol is unhealthy, and best avoided, because it can break the balance of emotional, physical, spiritual, and mental aspects of our health.

Canada's Food Guide to Healthy Eating

Suggests a range of daily servings for adults and children that include:

Grain Products:	**5-12 servings per day**
Examples of 1 serving:	1 slice of bread or bannock 3/4 cup of hot oatmeal
Vegetables and Fruit:	**5-10 servings per day**
Examples of 1 serving:	1 medium carrot 1/2 cup of juice 1/2 cup of canned fruit
Meat and Alternatives:	**2-3 servings per day**
Examples of 1 serving:	2/3 cup of canned fish 2 tbsp peanut butter 50-100 g caribou (a piece about the size of a deck of cards)
Milk Products:	**Servings per day for:** **Children ages 4-9 years:** 2-3 servings **Youth ages 10-16 years:** 3-4 servings **Adults:** 2-4 servings **Pregnant and breast feeding women:** 3-4 servings
Examples of 1 serving:	1 cup of milk 2 slices of processed cheese

The amount of food needed varies with each individual. A person's age, gender, and level of physical activity determine how many servings per day are needed for growth and development.

Example: A growing, active male teenager needs more food than an adult man who sits at a desk all day...

    OR

    A pregnant woman, or a breastfeeding mother needs more food than a non-pregnant, non-lactating woman of similar body size.

Recommendations:

1. Choose a **variety** of foods from each food group.

    Examples of **variety** include:
    - dark green, yellow, and red vegetables
    - edible roots, leaves, stems, and flowers of vegetables
    - fruit with different colours and textures
    - organs, bone marrow, and flesh of animals
    - bones, eggs, and flesh of fish
    - bannock, breads, pilot biscuits, hot and cold cereals, wild, brown, and converted white rice
    - preparing the same foods in different ways: apples, applesauce, dried apples, apple juice

* **Eating a variety of traditional and market foods contributes to a complete diet, which helps maintain good health.**

2. **"Energy in" should equal "energy out". This defines balance.**

    - **"Energy in"** is the energy from food which is eaten.
    - **"Energy out"** is the energy that is spent on everyday bodily functions and physical activity.
    - If **"Energy in"** is higher than **"Energy out"**, a person will gain weight.
    - Eating a balanced diet contributes to a balanced lifestyle and good health.

3. Eat foods in **moderation**.

    - Choosing only the amount of food that the body needs contributes to moderation.
    - Eat high fat/sugar foods only occasionally; they should not be a daily choice.
    - The amount of food that the body requires differs for each person according to age, gender, and level of physical activity.

4. **Dietary fibre** and **water** are important in the daily diet.

Nutrients for Our Body

What are nutrients?

Two main types of nutrients are macronutrients and micronutrients.

1. Macronutrients - provide energy.

a) **Protein - found in meat, fish, cheese, milk, beans, eggs, nuts, and seeds**

- helps build and repair body tissues
- helps fight infection
- supplies energy to the body

b) **Carbohydrates - found in bannock, berries, cereal, pasta, sugar, and roots**

- supply energy to the body
- help burn fat

c) **Fat - found in lard, butter, margarine, fatty meats, fish oils, vegetable oils, and salad dressings**

- supplies energy
- helps the body absorb vitamins A, D, E, K

2. Micronutrients - help the body use other nutrients

Micronutrients refer to vitamins and minerals in foods. Some important ones are:

a) **Calcium - found in milk, cheese, fish bones, yogurt, and bone soup**

- helps build strong bones and teeth
- helps blood clot when an injury occurs

b) **Folate - found in organ meat, dark green leafy vegetables, fruit, fish, eggs, nuts, and beans**

- helps make new cells
- helps make new red blood cells

c) **Vitamin A - found in deep orange-coloured vegetables such as carrots, turnips and squash, wild greens, moose and caribou liver, and in small amounts in milk and margarine**

- helps the body fight infection
- helps in maintaining healthy skin

d) **Vitamin D - found in fortified milk, salmon, eggs, margarine, fish and other livers**

- helps the body absorb calcium

e) **Vitamin C - found in berries, rose hips, fireweed leaves, oranges and other fruit, fruit juice, and certain fruit drink crystals (read the label.)**

- keeps teeth and gums healthy
- keeps blood vessel walls strong

Vitamin and Mineral Supplements

Choosing food wisely can generally provide all the required vitamins and minerals. However, there may be special times, such as during pregnancy or breastfeeding, when needs are especially high. Some people - often elders - have difficulty eating certain foods, and therefore may require supplements. Vitamin and mineral supplements should only be taken if recommended by a health professional.

3. Other Dietary Components

a) **Dietary Fibre - found in whole grain breads and bran cereals, legumes, fruits and vegetables which contain seeds or skins, such as berries and potato skins**

- helps prevent constipation
- helps maintain healthy blood sugar levels
- helps lower blood cholesterol levels
- since dietary fibre cannot be digested, it does not contribute energy

b) **Water**

- helps carry nutrients to the cells, and carry waste material away from the cells Throughout each day, the body loses water through sweating and urinating. It is important to replace fluid loss by drinking water, juice, and milk. Caffeinated beverages such as coffee, tea, and most pop cause the body to lose water; therefore, other fluids are better to drink.

Nutrients for Special Emphasis (Calcium, Fibre, Fat)

Calcium

What foods contain calcium?

1. Milk
2. Cheese
3. Soups or stews with bone
4. Yogurt
5. Fish head soup
6. Skim milk powder
7. Edible bones in canned fish (e.g., salmon or sardines)
8. Broccoli
9. Animal stomach contents
10. Dried beans/peas
11. Sunflower seeds

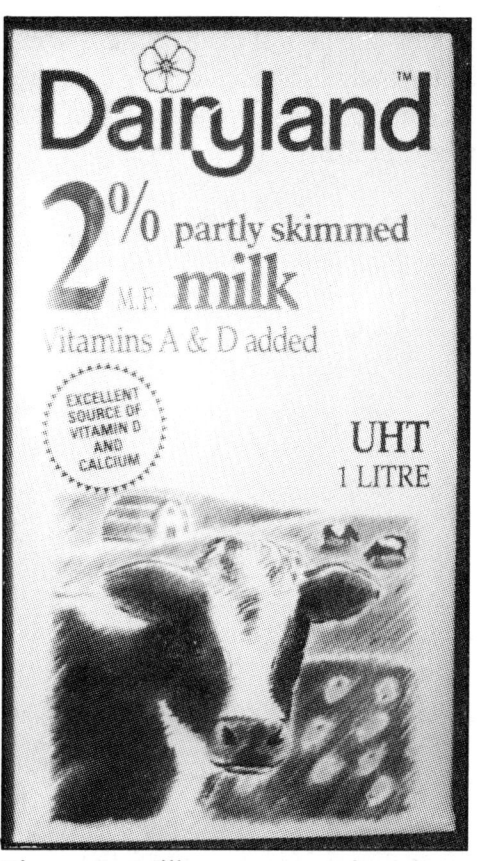

What does calcium do for our body?

1. Helps build strong bones and teeth

2. Helps build healthy nerves and promote blood clotting

Figure 7. Milk - a source of calcium, riboflavin, vitamins A and D (Photo: E.E. Wein).

What happens if we do not have enough calcium in our diet?

Sometimes as we get older, especially in women, bones may become thinner and bone mass decreases. This condition is called **osteoporosis**. A diet low in calcium may be a factor in the development of osteoporosis.

This condition may not have existed for Yukon First Nations people in the past, because their level of physical activity was much higher than it is now, and it is suspected that physical activity may help prevent the development of osteoporosis. Calcium sources in the traditional diet included mother's milk, bones of mammals and fish, and some fresh vegetables. Today, these traditional sources alone may not be sufficient to prevent osteoporosis.

Dietary Fibre

What is fibre?

Fibre is the part of plants (bran, oatmeal, berries, rhubarb etc.) that cannot be broken down by the body. This is "bulk" or "roughage". Fibre is classified as either **soluble** or **insoluble**. It is important to eat a variety of foods that contain fibre, including fruits, vegetables, and whole grains.

What foods contain fibre?

* Whole grain breads
* Whole grain cereals
* Bran muffins
* Legumes
* Berries
* Oatmeal
* Oranges
* Baked potato with skin
* Root vegetables
* Apples
* Bean salads
* Fireweed leaves
* Arctic dock
* Fruits and vegetables with seeds and skin

Why is fibre important? Fibre helps:

1. lower the level of fat in the blood.
2. lower cholesterol in the blood.
3. control blood sugar levels.
4. maintain a healthy digestive tract.
5. prevent constipation and reduce the risk of colon cancer.

The Two Rules of Fibre

1. Gradually increase the amount of dietary fibre. Too much fibre can cause minor bloating and gas which may feel uncomfortable.

2. Increase fluid intake as you increase the amount of high fibre foods in your diet. Fibre absorbs fluid in the digestive track and increases the amount of fluid needed.

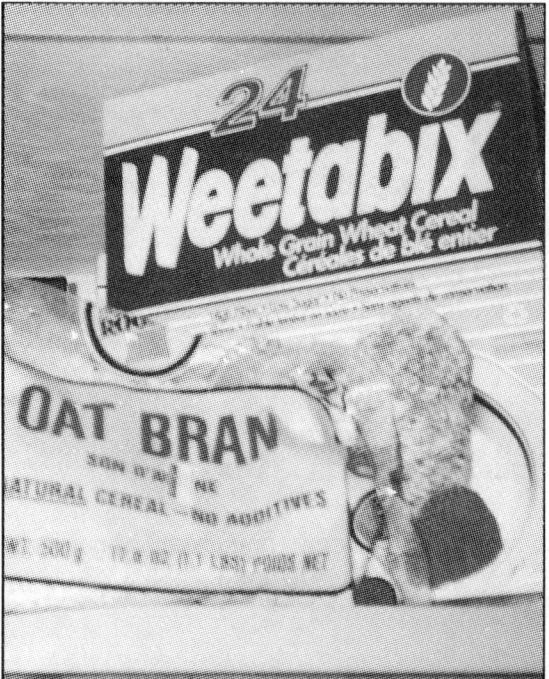

Figure 8. Whole grain cereals - a source of fibre (Photo: V. M. Nardelli).

Dietary Fat

What is cholesterol?

Cholesterol is a sticky or waxy fat-like substance made naturally by the body. In fact, most of the cholesterol found in the blood has been produced naturally, and only a small portion (about 20%) comes from food we eat. Cholesterol in food is called **dietary cholesterol**. Foods that contain dietary cholesterol include eggs, shell fish, organ meats, and animal fat.

It is important to limit dietary cholestrol. Cholesterol from food or produced by the body may build up along the walls of arteries and vessels that carry blood through the body. The effect is similar to the natural flow of a river which is slowed or blocked by a dam. Heart disease occurs when the vessels to the heart become clogged and the flow of blood is reduced.

What are the different types of fat, and what should we know about them?

1. **Saturated Fat:**

    - sources: animal fat such as lard, beef and moose fat, high-fat cheese, butter, cream, coconut, and palm oils
    - hard margarines (sold in a block, hard at refrigerator temperature) contain trans-fatty acids that affect the body in the same way as saturated fat.
    - **raises** blood cholesterol levels

2. **Polyunsaturated Fat:**

    - sources: fish, safflower, sunflower and corn oils, soft margarine, and some nuts such as almonds, filberts and walnuts
    - helps lower blood cholesterol

3. **Monounsaturated Fat:**

    - sources: olive, canola, and peanut oils
    - does not seem to influence blood cholesterol

4. **Omega-3 Fat:**

    - sources: fish oils, such as salmon
    - helps decrease the risk of heart disease

What is "total dietary fat"?

Total dietary fat is the sum of all types of fat contained in the food we eat. Including a variety of fat sources in **small amounts** contributes to a balanced diet. Limiting total dietary fat can help prevent heart disease and some cancers, and can lower blood cholesterol levels.

Low Fat Choices

Limit your daily intake of fats by choosing foods low in fat, and by using only small amounts or no added fat when preparing food.

Try some of these low-fat cooking ideas. Discuss new ideas with friends and family.

1. Prepare meat by broiling, boiling, roasting, barbequeing, or drying rather than frying.

2. Remove the skin from chicken, grouse, duck, and geese before eating.

3. Trim the visible fat off meat such as caribou, moose, pork, and beef.

4. When choosing milk, try skim, 1%, or 2% rather than whole or evaporated milk.

5. Use spices, herbs, vinegar, or lemon juice rather than butter, margarine, salad dressing, or lard.

6. When preparing soup or stew, remove some of the visible fat from the top after it cools.

7. Bake or boil potatoes, instead of frying them.

8. Bake bannock more often than frying it.

Food Safety

It is very important to practice safe storage, preparation, and cooking methods to avoid food poisoning. In fact, Public Health Regulations specify proper procedures to follow, especially in group situations, for cleaning anything (hands, utensils) used to prepare and/or serve foods. Symptoms of food poisoning include stomach ache, dizziness, vomiting, and diarrhea.

NOTE: A bleach mixture (9 parts water to 1 part bleach) is especially effective in reducing bacteria that cause food poisoning. **It must be used in all public eating places and at all occasions where several people are gathering to eat, including community feasts.**

Food Preparation:

Wash your hands thoroughly with warm soapy water before preparing food, and immediately after handling raw meat or fish. Thoroughly wash all utensils used to cut raw meat, fish and poultry. First wash with hot soapy water, then rinse with clean water, and then rinse a second time with the bleach mixture given above. Clean the work area, including the cutting boards, counters, and floors using the same method - wash with soapy water, rinse with water, then rinse again with the bleach mixture.

Food Storage:

Separate raw foods from prepared foods, to decrease the risk of cross-contamination (contaminating cooked foods with the germs from the raw foods). Refrigerate prepared foods containing eggs, meat, fish, or milk. Keep cooked foods hot (not just warm) until serving. Discard any food wrapping material, and use the bleach mixture to thoroughly clean any containers in which food has spoiled, in order to prevent cross-contamination. Check the expiry date on prepackaged meat, fish, and milk products before using.

Foods that can be especially harmful if they are not stored properly include:

* meat, fish, poultry
* milk products
* eggs
* ground meat, small cuts of meat found in stews
* hot dogs, bologna
* gravies and sauces
* unrefrigerated canned food which has been opened

Water Supply: Water that has not been taken directly from your own treated water supply should be boiled for at least 10 minutes before drinking. This will destroy any harmful bacteria (for example, the bacteria that causes "beaver fever").

SPECIAL DIETARY CONCERNS

The objectives of this section are:

1. To describe risk factors that contribute to **heart disease**.

2. To describe risk factors that contribute to **diabetes**.

3. To explain a condition called **lactose intolerance**.

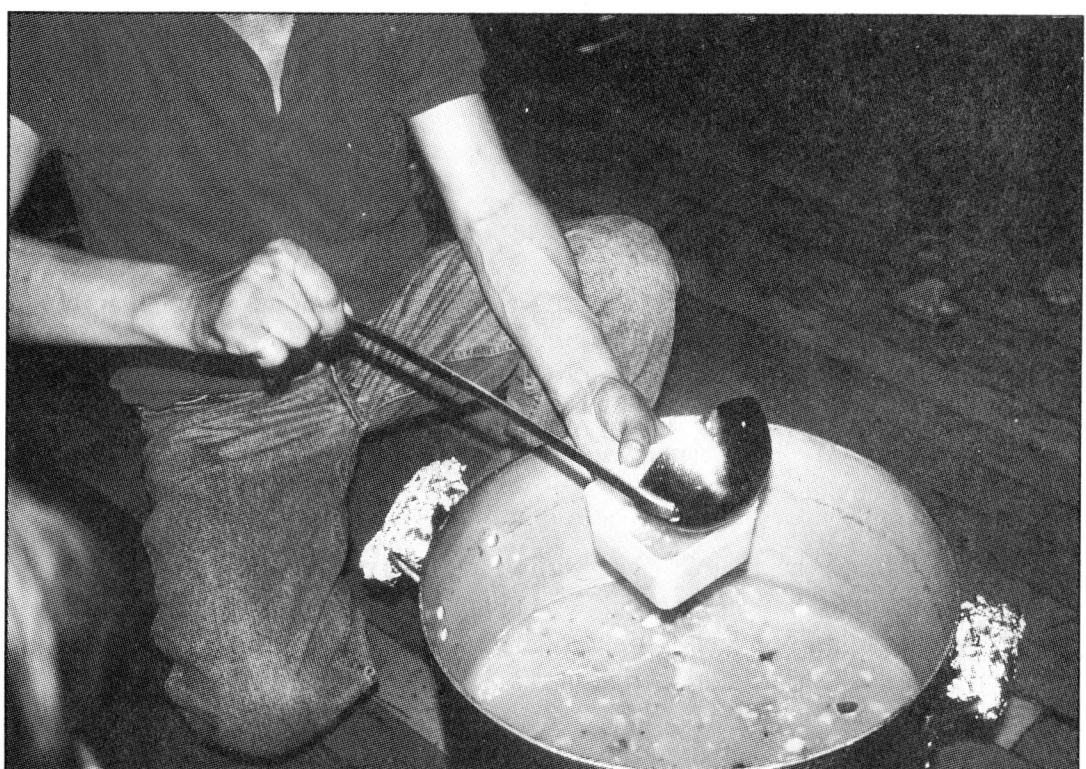

Figure 9. Moose head soup served at a feast in Old Crow (Photo: E.E.Wein).

Heart Disease

What is Heart Disease?

Heart disease is a condition that involves a restricted flow of blood to the heart.

Heart disease may develop under several conditions:

1. **Heredity** - many members of the same family may develop heart disease

2. **Obesity** - a condition of excessive overweight
   (example: more than 10 kilograms above healthy weight)

3. **Stress** - physical, emotional, spiritual or mental exhaustion

4. **Smoking**

5. **Inactive lifestyle**

6. **High blood cholesterol**

How can we decrease our risk of developing heart disease?

1. Maintain a healthy body weight by eating a variety of traditional and market foods that are low in fat and sugar, high in fibre, and contain many nutrients.

2. Maintain a moderate level of physical activity by doing something active at least three times a week. Walking, playing sports, hunting, fishing, and berry picking are examples of activities.

Individuals with high blood cholesterol or **heart disease** should choose foods that are low in total fat, especially saturated fat (e.g., fish and lean cuts of meat). Foods that are high in fibre (e.g., berries, whole grains, vegetables) are also important. Salt intake may increase blood pressure, which makes the heart work harder, and so should be limited in the diet.

Obesity increases the risk not only of heart disease, but of many other conditions, such as diabetes and some cancers. Fast weight loss diets are not a reasonable solution; however, healthy eating and increased physical activity can help in achieving and maintaining a healthy weight.

Diabetes Mellitus

What is Diabetes?

Diabetes is a condition that occurs when the body does not produce enough insulin, a substance that helps blood sugar get absorbed into cells. Cells require sugar that can be converted to fuel, which provides energy. Without insulin, the body cells can "starve", while levels of sugar in the blood rise. Diabetes symptoms can be controlled with a healthy diet and regular physical activity. Sometimes, medication is required. It is important to remember, however, that a person with diabetes can live a comfortable and healthy life.

Three types of diabetes include:

a) **Insulin Dependent** - The body does **not produce any** insulin. Insulin injections are required to control blood sugar levels.

b) **Non-Insulin Dependent** - The body does **not produce enough** insulin, or the insulin does not work properly. (This is the most common type among aboriginal people.) Diet alone, with pills, or with insulin, and exercise are needed to control blood sugar levels. Eating a balanced diet, maintaining a healthy body weight, being physically active, and coping well with stress, may help prevent the development of diabetes, especially the non-insulin dependent type.

c) **Gestational** - This type of diabetes can develop during pregnancy, but is not always permanent. Blood sugar must be controlled during pregnancy, since high blood sugar can harm the baby. The baby is not necessarily born with diabetes, but is at greater risk of developing diabetes later in life; the mother is also at risk.

In all types of diabetes, it is important to control daily blood sugar levels, in order to feel well and to prevent complications from developing in the future.

What are the symptoms of diabetes?

- hungrier than usual
- thirstier than usual
- urinating more often
- more tired than usual
- undesired weight loss

Note: Anyone who develops two or more of these symtoms should see a doctor.

Dietary Needs: Choose a variety of traditional and market foods that provide many nutrients and little fat. Include fruits, vegetables, whole grain breads and cereals. A regular daily pattern of food and activity will help maintain healthy body weight and control the symptoms of diabetes. Alcoholic beverages should be avoided: they are low in nutrients and some contain sugar, as well as alcohol.

Lactose Intolerance

What is Lactose Intolerance?

Lactose is a natural sugar found in milk. A person who has **Lactose Intolerance** cannot digest lactose, and so will suffer from stomach cramps and diarrhea after consuming milk. Depending on the severity of the condition, the person may be able to tolerate small amounts of milk or milk products without feeling sick.

How can a person with lactose intolerance ensure that they get calcium in their diet?

It is important that a person with lactose intolerance eat other foods that contain calcium, such as fish heads and bones, seeds, bone soups, and canned fish with edible bones (for example, canned salmon or sardines). Cheese and yogurt can usually be tolerated, because the amount of lactose in these products has been reduced through processing. Ice cream and chocolate milk may be tolerated by some individuals, especially in moderate amounts. Calcium supplements can be helpful for those who are extremely lactose intolerant, but a doctor or nutritionist should be consulted first.

Some special medicinal products are available to help with this condition. **Lactaid™** tablets can be taken with regular milk or meals to help with digestion. **Lacteeze™** products are also available, which are milk products that have already been treated to reduce the lactose content. Unfotunately, Lacteeze™ products are generally more expensive than regular milk. Some people find cultured products helpful, such as acidophilus milk, available at most large grocery stores.

SPECIAL NEEDS THROUGH THE LIFECYCLE

The objectives of this section are:

1. To describe some **special dietary needs during pregnancy**.

2. To provide information about **breastfeeding**.

3. To provide information about **formula feeding**.

4. To describe ways of **introducing solid foods to infants**.

5. To describe some **special dietary needs of the elderly**.

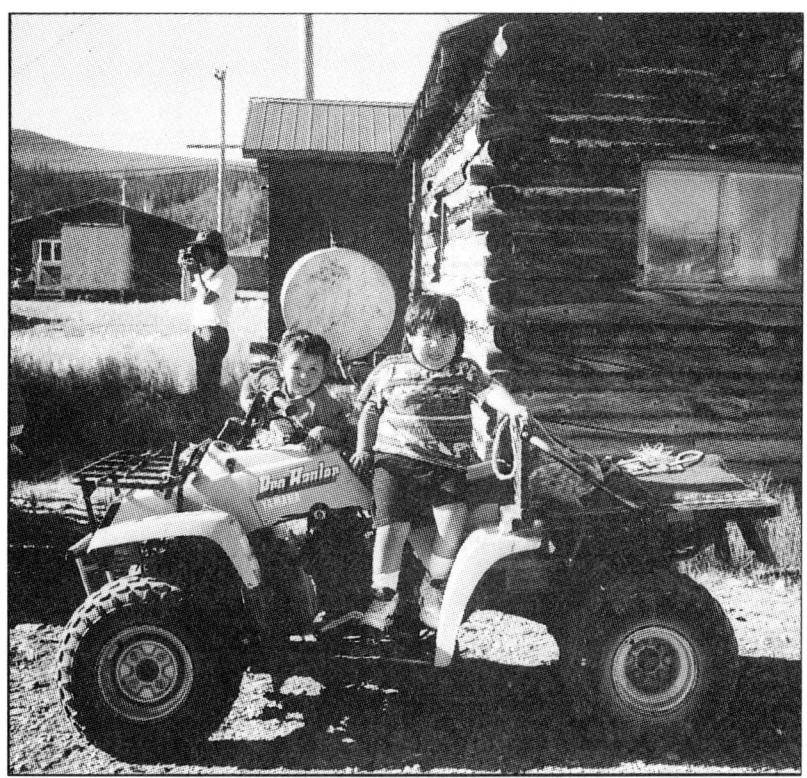

Figure 10. Children in Old Crow (Photo: V.M.Nardelli).

Pregnancy

Throughout pregnancy, a woman's body requires more nutrients and energy to build the tissues that support the baby in the womb, and to build up nutrient stores in preparation for breastfeeding. Healthy food choices will provide both mother and baby with the nutrients required for growth and development.

A pregnant teenager has an even greater challenge with respect to food intake. The teen's body is still developing, so she needs a diet rich in nutrients. She must provide both her body and the baby with enough nutrients and energy for growth and development.

Increasing fluid intake such as fruit juice, milk, and water is also important, as they help deliver nutrients to the baby and carry waste products away.

Pregnant women should wait no longer than four hours between meals. Smaller meals and snacks should be eaten more often, even though the mother may not feel hungry, since the baby still requires sufficient nourishment.

What do some nutrients do for my baby?

a) **Protein**
- helps build blood, nerve, muscle, and brain cells
- helps build stores for labour, delivery, and breastfeeding

b) **Iron** - helps produce red blood cells

c) **Calcium**
- helps strengthen bones and teeth
- helps build reserves for breastfeeding

d) **Vitamin A** - helps develop healthy skin and membranes

e) **Vitamin C** - helps strengthen gums, blood vessels, bones, and teeth

f) **Vitamin D** - works with calcium to build strong bones and teeth

g) **Folate** - helps produce healthy red and white blood cells

h) **B Vitamins (thiamin, riboflavin, niacin)**
- help promote normal appetite and build healthy skin and nerves

Most nutrients can be obtained from a balanced diet. However, with an increased need for nutrients during pregnancy, many health professionals recommend certain vitamin supplements, particularly folate (Canadian Dietetic Association 1995). Furthermore, in northern native communities where exposure to sunlight is limited, and milk is often not a staple of the diet, supplemental vitamin D is usually recommended during pregnancy, breastfeeding, and through the winter months (Canadian Paediatric Society 1988). Consult a health professional for advice about the type and amount of supplement(s) you may require during your pregnancy.

Special Considerations:

a) **Alcohol** - Intake at any time during pregnancy can have negative effects on the fetus and may cause **Fetal Alcohol Syndrome (FAS).** Some major consequences of FAS are fetal growth deficiency, abnormal facial characteristics, and mental retardation.

b) **Smoking** - Smoking blocks the blood supply of nutrients to the fetus, and harms the baby's growth and development.

c) **Caffeine** - Products containing caffeine such as coffee, tea, soft drinks, chocolate, and some medications should be consumed in moderation, if at all. A "recommended maximum" level of caffeine intake during pregnancy has not yet been established; therefore, it is best to have as little as possible.

d) **Aspartame** - Many "lite" or "diet" products contain sugar replacements such as aspartame. Such products are intended for weight loss, which should not be attempted during pregnancy. A "recommended maximum" level of aspartame intake during pregnancy has not yet been established; therefore, it is best to have as little as possible.

Infant Feeding

Breastfeeding

Breastfeeding is a wonderful experience shared between mother and child. It is a convenient and natural way to feed a baby. Breast milk is the ideal source of food for a baby because it contains many nutrients necessary for growth and development. The colostrum (early secretion in the first few days after birth, before the mature milk) contains antibodies that help protect the baby against infection. This benefit is unique to breastfeeding.

The following remarks answer a few common questions about breastfeeding.

a) **Drugs, alcohol and smoking adversely affect breast milk.**

- Some drugs such as aspirin, laxatives, tranquilizers, and cough medicines pass to the baby through breast milk.

- Alcohol and caffeine pass from breast milk to the baby.

- Nicotine from smoking passes through breast milk to the baby, and can cause stomach cramps and vomiting.

b) **The more often a baby is fed, the more milk is produced.**

- As the baby grows and takes more milk, the mother's body produces more to accommodate the growing need.

- Breast milk is the only food that a baby needs for about the first six months.

c) **The mother's diet affects the quality of her breast milk.**

- An insufficient diet may result in low milk production.

- A diet severely lacking in nutrients can lower the nutrient quality of the breast milk, although it usually does not affect its energy (calorie) content.

d) **Extra fluids are needed while breastfeeding.**

- More water, juice, and milk are needed to produce sufficient quantities of breast milk.

e) **Supplements of vitamin D are recommended.**

The Canadian Paediatric Society (1988) recommends that in northern native communities, both nursing mothers and their breastfed infants should take supplemental vitamin D. The skin produces some vitamin D when exposed to sunlight; however, in the far north, the lack of daylight in winter, and the protective clothing required against insects in summer reduce the amount of vitamin D produced this way; hence, special recommendations apply to northern mothers and infants.

f) **The mother should take extra good care of herself.**

- Pregnancy, childbirth, and breastfeeding require a great deal of energy; therefore, it is important to get sufficient rest.

- The natural weight gain of pregnancy provides a reserve for the even greater energy demands of lactation. The extra energy required to produce breastmilk for several months and to care for the baby usually helps the mother lose the weight she gained during pregancy. This natural process is another benefit of breastfeeding, and so weight loss diets are not needed, nor are they recommended, during this time.

- Breast milk can be expressed into a bottle so that the father or other family member can feed the baby occasionally.

g) **Weaning a baby can be accomplished between age 6 months and 1 year.**

- Replace one breastfeeding per day with a cup for a few days, then replace a second feeding per day for a few more days, etc., until the infant gradually is comfortable with the new feeding method. As breastfeeding becomes less frequent, the mother's milk supply will gradually decrease.

Important: Avoid giving a bottle of milk or juice to the baby as he/she is falling asleep, because this may cause tooth decay in the front teeth.

Formula Feeding

Why feed with formula?

Breast milk is the ideal food, and breastfeeding the ideal method of feeding; it is also convenient and economical. Most mothers can produce enough milk for their babies, especially if the baby is fed as often as he/she demands. Only when there are valid reasons to avoid breastfeeding (such as alcohol consumption, illicit drug use, failure to thrive), should formula feeding be considered.

Prepared Formula is the best type.

Many types of prepared formula are available, including ready-to-use and powdered formulas. Prepared formulas have been designed to be as close as possible to breast milk. It is important to prepare formula correctly for reasons of safety and nutrient value. Follow package instructions closely. Formula should never be made more dilute than the package directs, as the infant will not get enough energy and nutrients.

A mother who has decided to breastfeed should not use formula at an early stage, because this will decrease production of breast milk. However, after breastfeeding is well established (e.g. after two months), formula can be used as an occasional alternative. Using formula too frequently, however, will decrease the mother's own milk supply.

For more information about formula feeding, ask a nurse or health educator.

Home-made Formula - a last resort.

As a last resort, when neither breastfeeding nor purchasing prepared formula is possible, a formula can be made with evaporated milk. This type is the least like mother's natural milk.

Formula made with **evaporated milk**: (Reference: Medical Services Branch 1994)

	Age 0-6 months	Age 7-12 months
Quantity of formula to make	**1200 mL**	**800 mL**
Evaporated whole milk	400 mL	400 mL
Cooled boiled water	800 mL	400 mL
Sugar	60 mL	

Instructions:

1. Sterilize all utensils first in boiling water for 5-10 minutes.

2. Boil 800 mL of water in a covered sauce pan 10 minutes (for infants 0-6 months). Remove from heat and add sugar. Open a fresh 14 oz (400mL) can of regular evaporated milk (not 2%) and pour directly into the sauce pan. With sterilized spoon, stir the mixture. (For infants 7-12 months, use 400 mL water with one can of milk, and no sugar).

3. Pour formula into 5 large or 10 small sterilized baby bottles and refrigerate. Prior to feeding, place one bottle into hot water until the formula is lukewarm. Pretest the formula on your wrist to ensure that it is not too hot.

4. Discard any formula remaining in the bottle after the baby has finished eating.

Introducing Solid Foods to Infants

After 4 months of age, small amounts of soft-textured foods can be introduced, such as oatmeal, stewed fruits, soft mashed vegetables, and eventually small tender cuts of chicken or meat, along with continued breast milk or formula. Learning to eat from a spoon and to move solid food to the back of the mouth before swallowing is a new experience for a baby. In addition, infants have small stomachs; therefore, they need to eat small portions more often throughout the day.

Ages 4 to 6 months:

- infant cereals with added iron
- plain mashed vegetables (squash, peas, green/yellow beans)
- plain mashed fruit (bananas, applesauce)

Ages 7 to 9 months:

- increase mashed green, yellow, and orange-coloured vegetables and fruits, since colourful foods will tempt a child's curiosity.
- cooked cereals, oatmeal, rice, noodles, and bannock
- soft-cooked finely cut poultry and mashed fish without the bones

Ages 10 to 12 months

- use whole (homogenized) milk rather than low fat milk in the first year
- offer fruit juice once the infant can drink from a cup
- avoid spicy foods and sauces
- egg white can be fed at 12 months of age, but may cause allergies if given earlier
- avoid foods that may cause choking, such as nuts, seeds, popcorn, chips, and dry cereals

Older infants need a variety of traditional and market foods for growth. Foods that contain fat, sugar, or salt should be given infrequently and in small amounts. Foods containing alcohol or caffeine should not be given to infants.

If there is concern about a child being overweight, talk to a health professional. Children should not worry about weight-loss diets. They should eat a variety of healthy foods and be physically active.

If a child appears to be underweight and not growing normally, talk to a doctor or nurse. Try offering more snacks, such as dried salmon and pilot biscuits, or dried caribou or moose. A child should never feel hungry for any length of time.

Elders

As people get older, their food habits may change. Loss of appetite, lower taste sensation, and chewing and swallowing difficulties may alter food choices for elders. In addition, some medications, such as diuretics, laxatives and antacids, cause some nutrients to be "washed out" of the body before they have been absorbed.

Nutrition for the Elderly

1. **Fluids** - Water, juice, milk, and soups provide nutrients and help prevent dehydration that can be caused by medications, or diarrhea, etc.

2. **Fibre** - Elders need foods that contain fibre, that will help prevent constipation. Many fresh vegetables and fruits are firm and fibrous, which make them difficult for elders to chew. Oatmeal, cooked fruit and vegetables are easier to eat, and provide fibre and other nutrients.

3. **Protein** - Protein is important for tissue repair.

4. **Calcium** - As a person gets older, bone mass decreases. Calcium helps strengthen bones. Women in particular, and especially after menopause, are at greater risk of developing osteoporosis. Post-menopausal women and elders, therefore, should eat foods containing calcium such as fish heads and bones, canned fish with edible bones, or milk products. Lacteeze™ milk can be added to soups as a calcium supplement as well.

5. **Fat** - Eating too many foods that are high in fat can cause a person to become overweight. As age increases, the risk of developing heart disease and diabetes increases, and being overweight can contribute to both diseases.

6. **Vitamin A** - Dark green and yellow vegetables such as beans, spinach, carrots, squash, turnip and arctic dock contain vitamin A. These vegetables may be more palatable for elders if they are cooked, or softened in some way for easier eating. Vegetables should also be added to soups and stews (choose a variety for colour, flavour, and nutrients).

7. **Vitamin C** - Many citrus fruits such as oranges, grapefruit, tomatoes, and berries such as strawberries, cranberries, and rosehips contain vitamin C. Stewed fruits and fruit juices may be more appropriate for those who have difficulty chewing or swallowing.

Making Food Easier to Eat

If someone has difficulty chewing and/or swallowing, try the following to make foods easier to eat.

1. **Meat Products**

    - Cook moose and caribou in stews, or boil or roast meat to make it more tender.
    - Grind moose and caribou, or cut the meat into fine strips.
    - Can fish.
    - Boil grouse, duck, or geese.

2. **Vegetables and Fruit**

    - Can, stew, or steam vegetables and fruit such as berries, beans, tomatoes, and rhubarb.
    - Mash potatoes, turnips, carrots, and squash.
    - Chop vegetables into bite-size pieces and cook well.
    - Make vegetable soup, or add vegetables to stew, tomato sauce, or chili.
    - Serve fruit juice.

3. **Grain Products**

    - Cook oatmeal, cornmeal, cream of wheat, and porridge
    - Cook rice or barley until very tender
    - Add rice or barley to soups and stews or pasta (e.g., macaroni) to soups and stews.

4. **Milk Products**

    - Add grated cheese to salads or sandwiches.
    - Melt cheese on bannock.
    - Serve milkshakes as a good source of calcium.
    - Serve ice cream or yogurt for dessert.

Encourage elders to share ideas about their favourite foods, or foods that they find easy to eat.

Summary of points to mention:

1. Many elders do not eat enough food, or the proper or healthy foods that provide enough nutrients. A lack of taste or difficulties chewing and/or swallowing certain foods may be contributing to these habits. Although simple foods such as tea and bannock may satisfy hunger, they do not provide enough nutrients for a healthy, balanced diet.

2. In order to provide the body with enough energy and nutrients for activities such as cooking, gardening, berry picking, and playing with grandchildren, it is important to eat a variety of foods from the four major food groups.

GAMES AND ACTIVITIES

The objective of this section is to provide "hands on" activities that will improve awareness and understanding of good food and nutrition practices.

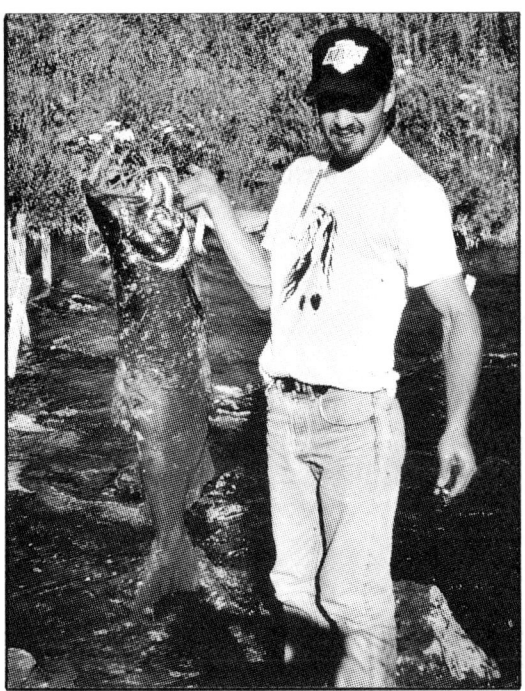

Figure 11. Daniel Green with a salmon he caught at Klukshu.
(Photo: V.M. Nardelli)

Food Group Photo Game

Objective: To illustrate the four major food groups using traditional and market foods.

Materials:
- pencils or crayons
- poster paper
- ruler
- magazine or advertising flyers with food pictures
- glue

Activity:

1. Discuss the four food groups, providing examples of foods in each group.

2. Encourage participants to draw pictures of their favourite traditional foods.

3. Examples of market foods can be cut from the magazines or flyers provided.

4. Divide a large sheet of paper into four sections, listing one of the major food groups in each:

    a) Milk and Calcium Products
    b) Meat and Alternatives
    c) Grain Products
    d) Vegetables and Fruit

5. Group the magazine and hand-drawn pictures according to the four major food groups under the appropriate section on the poster. Compare the group poster to the food guide provided in Appendix I (p. 71-72) of this handbook.

6. Use the **Food Group Review** form as a tool to evaluate knowledge. Use the **General Evaluation** sheet (p. 67) to evaluate interest level and presentation of the topic.

Summary of points to mention:

1. Eat foods from each of the four food groups every day.
2. Include foods with different colours and textures to ensure variety.
3. Eat food in moderation; this will contribute to balance in the diet.

Variety + Balance + Moderation = Healthy Eating

Food Group Review

1. What are the four food groups?
2. Give three examples of recommended foods in each group. Include traditional foods as much as possible.

Food Group 1. _____ Example 1. _____

　　　　　　　　　　　　　　　　　　Example 2. _____

　　　　　　　　　　　　　　　　　　Example 3. _____

Food Group 2. _____ Example 1. _____

　　　　　　　　　　　　　　　　　　Example 2. _____

　　　　　　　　　　　　　　　　　　Example 3. _____

Food Group 3. _____ Example 1. _____

　　　　　　　　　　　　　　　　　　Example 2. _____

　　　　　　　　　　　　　　　　　　Example 3. _____

Food Group 4. _____ Example 1. _____

　　　　　　　　　　　　　　　　　　Example 2. _____

　　　　　　　　　　　　　　　　　　Example 3. _____

3. _____ + _____ + _____ = **Healthy Eating**

Nutrient Bingo

Objective: **To increase awareness of the nutrient content of some traditional and market foods.**

Materials:
- Bingo markers (use household items such as dried beans, buttons, or pennies)
- Prize for winners (Examples: box of cereal, bag of potatoes, oranges, apples, turnip, canned or powdered or UHT milk, can of beans, corn, peaches).

Activity:

1. Make copies of each of the five bingo cards in the book. The **Master Card** is used by the instructor, educator, or group leader. Distribute bingo cards to each player.

2. Each player should have at least 20 bingo markers. The educator should have at least 36.

3. Make a copy of the "**Bingo Game Sheet**" (next page). Cut out squares and place the paper pieces into a container or jar. Randomly select one piece of paper and read it to the group: Example: "Under Vitamin C, Oranges". Players are to place a bingo marker in the box on their card having that item.

4. Continue calling out the categories, as in a regular bingo game. When a diagonal or horizontal row is filled, the winning player has a "BINGO". Diagonal or horizontal lines represent variety in the diet. Continue the game until all the prizes have been given out. Keep the cards to reuse them for future games.

5. Distribute a copy of the **Bingo Handout** (page 45) that summarizes the functions and sources of the nutrients discussed.

6. Have copies of the **Fireweed Potato Salad** recipe (page 44) available for interested participants.

BINGO GAME SHEET

Instructions: Cut out and place labelled squares into an empty jar or container. Select one square at a time and call out the category. (eg: "Under Vitamin C, Oranges")

Vitamin C	Fibre	Vitamin A	Calcium	Vitamin D	Folate
Oranges	Blue-berries	Carrots	Milk	Fish Eggs	Spinach
Bear Root	Oatmeal	Caribou Liver	Sunflower Seeds	Milk	Oranges
Rosehips	Beans	Moose Liver	Fish Heads and Bones	Margarine	Cabbage
Fireweed Leaves	Whole Wheat Bannock	Dandelion Leaves	Cheese	Salmon	Beans
Cran-berries	Black-berries	Milk	Ice Cream	Moose Liver	Swiss Chard
Straw-berries	Apples	Corn	Chocolate Milk	Bird Eggs	Beets

Bingo Master Card

VITAMIN C	FIBRE	VITAMIN A	CALCIUM	VITAMIN D	FOLATE
Oranges	Blue-berries	Carrots	Milk	Fish Eggs	Spinach
Bear Root	Oatmeal	Caribou Liver	Sunflower Seeds	Milk	Oranges
Rosehips	Beans	Moose Liver	Fish Head and Bones	Margarine	Cabbage
Fireweed Leaves	Whole Wheat Bannock	Dandelion Leaves	Cheese	Salmon	Beans
Cran-berries	Black Berries	Milk	Ice Cream	Moose Liver	Swiss Chard
Straw-berries	Apples	Corn	Chocolate Milk	Bird Eggs	Beets

Summary of points to mention:

1. Many foods can be found under more than one nutrient heading, illustrating that many foods contain more than one important nutrient and some foods share common nutrients.

2. When choosing foods, keep in mind that a variety of food sources provide the body with nutrients needed for growth, development, and energy.

3. Remember that all nutrients depend on each other - they work together. If one nutrient is missing or too limited in the diet, this will affect the work of the others. This is another reason why a variety of foods is so important for good health.

Card #1

VIT. C	FIBRE	VIT. A	CALCIUM	VIT. D	FOLATE
Cranberries	Whole Wheat Bannock	Caribou Liver	Ice Cream	Moose Liver	Beets
Oranges	Beans	Milk	Sunflower Seeds	Fish Eggs	Swiss Chard
Rosehips	Apples	Carrots	Milk	Milk	Oranges
Fireweed Leaves	Oatmeal	Moose Liver	Cheese	Salmon	Spinach
Bear Root	Blueberries	Dandelion Leaves	Fish Head and Bones	Margarine	Cabbage

Card #2

VIT. C	FIBRE	VIT. A	CALCIUM	VIT. D	FOLATE
Rosehips	Beans	Moose Liver	Cheese	Margarine	Cabbage
Strawberries	Oatmeal	Carrots	Fish Head and Bones	Salmon	Spinach
Bear Root	Whole Wheat Bannock	Milk	Ice Cream	Bird Eggs	Beans
Cranberries	Blackberries	Caribou Liver	Milk	Fish Eggs	Oranges
Fireweed Leaves	Blueberries	Fireweed Leaves	Sunflower Seeds	Moose Liver	Swiss Chard

Card #3

VIT. C	FIBRE	VIT. A	CALCIUM	VIT. D	FOLATE
Rosehips	Blackberries	Milk	Sunflower Seeds	Salmon	Swiss Chard
Fireweed Leaves	Blueberries	Moose Liver	Milk	Moose Liver	Beans
Cranberries	Oatmeal	Carrots	Fish Head and Bones	Fish Eggs	Spinach
Bear Root	Beans	Corn	Ice Cream	Milk	Cabbage
Oranges	Whole Wheat Bannock	Caribou Liver	Cheese	Margarine	Oranges

Card #4

VIT. C	FIBRE	VIT. A	CALCIUM	VIT. D	FOLATE
Fireweed Leaves	Whole Wheat Bannock	Dandelion Leaves	Fish Head and Bones	Milk	Salmon
Cranberries	Blackberries	Moose Liver	Cheese	Margarine	Moose Liver
Oranges	Oatmeal	Milk	Sunflower Seeds	Salmon	Spinach
Bear Root	Blueberries	Caribou Liver	Milk	Fish Eggs	Caribou Liver
Rosehips	Rhubarb	Carrots	Chocolate Milk	Moose Liver	Beans

Card #5

VIT. C	FIBRE	VIT. A	CALCIUM	VIT. D	FOLATE
Bear Root	Whole Wheat Oatmeal	Carrots	Milk	Fish Eggs	Spinach
Rosehips	Bannock	Dandelion Leaves	Ice Cream	Milk	Cabbage
Fireweed Leaves	Blackberries	Moose Liver	Sunflower Seeds	Bird Eggs	Swiss Chard
Oranges	Blueberries	Milk	Cheese	Moose Liver	Beets
Cranberries	Beans	Caribou Liver	Fish Head and Bones	Salmon	Oranges

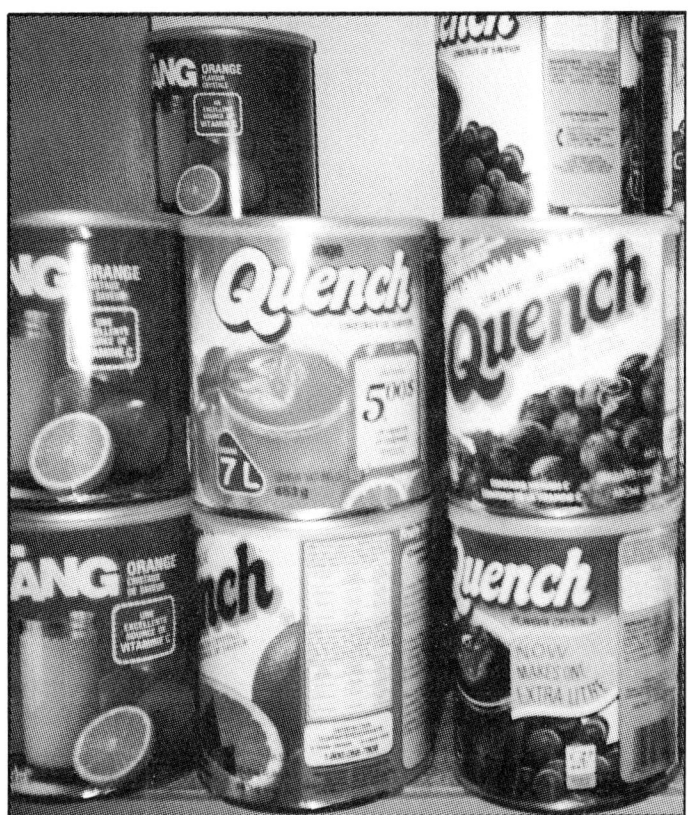

Figure 12. Only some brands of fruit crystals contain vitamin C. Check the label (Photo: V.M. Nardelli)

Fireweed Potato Salad

1/2 cup	fireweed leaves	125 mL
3 cups	diced potatoes	750 mL
3/4 cup	plain yogurt	175 mL
1/2 cup	mayonnaise	125 mL
1/2 cup	chopped celery	125 mL
1/4 cup	diced green pepper	60 mL
1 tsp	dry dill	5 mL
1 tsp	parsley flakes	5 mL

1. Boil the potatoes until cooked and allow to cool.

2. Cut the potatoes into bite sized cubes.

3. Mix yogurt, mayonnaise, dill, and parsley.

4. Add potatoes, fireweed leaves, celery, and green pepper.

5. Refrigerate until ready to serve.

Adapted from: Walker 1984

Bingo Handout

Post this chart on your refrigerator so that your family can see the functions and food sources of nutrients that their bodies need.

Eat foods that have high nutrient value, using this chart as a guide. Add other fruits, vegetables, whole grain breads and cereals, milk, lean meat, and fish for variety.

VITAMIN C	FIBRE	VITAMIN A	CALCIUM	VITAMIN D	FOLATE
- keeps teeth & gums healthy	-prevents constipation -maintains blood sugar levels	-fights infection -maintains vision	- builds bones & teeth - helps blood clot	- helps absorb calcium	- helps make new red blood cells
Bear Root	Oatmeal	Caribou Liver	Sunflower Seeds	Milk	Oranges
Rosehips	Beans	Moose Liver	Fish Head and Bones	Margarine	Cabbage
Fireweed Leaves	Whole Wheat Bannock	Dandelion Leaves	Cheese	Salmon	Beans
Cran-berries	Black-berries	Milk	Ice Cream	Moose Liver	Swiss Chard
Straw-berries	Apples	Corn	Chocolate Milk	Bird Eggs	Beets
Oranges	Blue-berries	Carrots	Milk	Fish Eggs	Spinach

Calcium Tips

Objective: To increase understanding of the role of calcium and its food sources.

Materials: none

Activity:

1. Discuss market foods that contain calcium.
2. Discuss traditional foods that contain calcium.
3. Discuss how calcium can be added to favourite dishes.
4. See below for other ideas to share. The recipes can be copied as handouts.

Adding Calcium To Our Meal Can Be Easy!

1. Use liquid or powdered milk instead of water when making bannock or doughnuts.

2. Add milk to canned soup instead of water.

3. Add milk to macaroni and cheese dinner.

4. Use milk or powdered milk in coffee instead of whitener.

5. Melt cheese over steamed vegetables.

6. Add a slice of cheese to pilot biscuits.

7. Eat the bones of canned fish.

8. Add sunflower seeds to cooked oatmeal.

9. Choose chocolate milk instead of pop.

10. Try hot cocoa made with milk instead of water.

11. Add milk or powdered milk to mashed potatoes.

12. Add grated cheese to pastas, casseroles or salads.

13. Add milk to rice pudding.

14. Choose yogurt or ice cream for dessert or a snack.

Cooking with Calcium

Quick and Easy Casserole

3/4 cup	brown rice	175 mL
2 cups	water	500 mL
1 cup	plain yogurt	250 mL
1 cup	shredded Mozzarella cheese	250 mL
1/2 cup	2% cottage cheese	125 mL
1/2 cup	chopped onion	125 mL
1/4 cup	chopped mushrooms	50 mL
1/4 cup	chopped green pepper	50 mL
1/4 tsp.	salt	1 mL
1/4 tsp.	ground pepper	1 mL
1/2 tsp.	garlic chopped	2 mL

1. Boil rice in a pot. Cover and cook at a low temperature until tender. Set aside.

2. While the rice is hot, stir in the yogurt, mozzarella and cottage cheese, onion, mushrooms, green pepper, garlic, salt, and pepper.

3. Put the mixture into a lightly greased casserole dish. Cook for 25 minutes, uncovered in a 350°F (180°C) oven. Makes 6 servings.

Adapted from: Bishop-MacDonald and Howard 1990

My Favourite Salmon Chowder

1 pound	salmon or other fish	500 g
1/2 cup	chopped carrots	125 mL
1/3 cup	chopped onion	75 mL
1/3 cup	chopped red pepper	75 mL
2 cups	diced potatoes	500 mL
2/3 cup	water	150 mL
2 tsp	salt	10 mL
3 cups	milk	750 mL
1 1/2 cup	corn	375 mL
3 tbsp	flour	45 mL
1 1/4 cup	evaporated milk	300 mL
1/2 tsp	pepper	2 mL
1 tbsp	margarine	15 mL
1 tbsp	parsley	15 mL

1. Cut fish into small pieces.

2. Saute onion in margarine in a large sauce pan.

3. Add potatoes, carrots, red pepper, fish, water, and salt. Bring to a boil.

4. Reduce heat and cover until potatoes and fish are tender. Stir in milk and corn.

5. Combine flour and evaporated milk before adding to mixture. Cook over medium heat and stir until mixture just comes to a boil and thickens. Makes about 7 1/2 cups (1.75 L)

Adapted from: Ontario Milk Marketing Board 1990

Fibre Everyday!

Objective: To increase awareness of the role of fibre and its sources in order to increase dietary intake of fibre.

Materials: none

Activity:

1. Discuss traditional and market foods that are good sources of fibre.

2. Discuss how fibre can be added to the diet using both traditional and market foods.

3. **"Making Fibre a Part of Every Meal"** (next page) includes tips on how to increase fibre in meals or snacks. This sheet and the recipes on the pages that follow can be copied as handouts.

4. Use the **Fibre Review** form and the **General Evaluation** (p. 67) to evaluate what was learned.

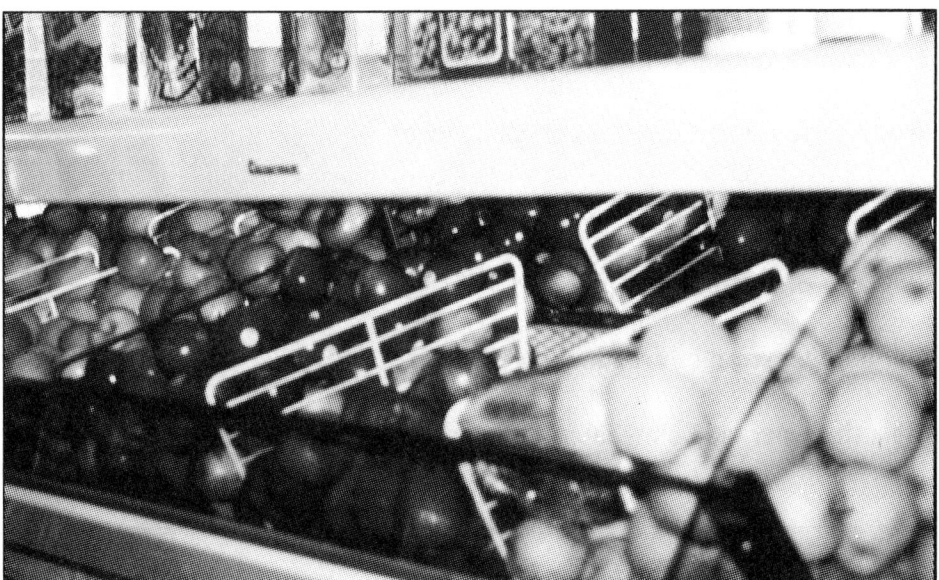

Figure 13. Fresh fruit provides some fibre along with vitamin C. A variety of fresh fruit is available at the Nisutlin Trading Post in Teslin. (Photo: E.E. Wein).

Making Fibre a Part of Every Meal

1. Add dried berries, oatmeal, and/or bran to bannock.

2. Replace half of the flour for bannock with whole wheat flour, bran or oatmeal.

3. Add grated carrots or apples to muffins or bannock.

4. Crumble a handful of bran flake cereal or rolled oats on top of casseroles, pasta or macaroni and cheese dinners.

5. Add cooked vegetables to spaghetti sauce.

6. Have an apple slice with a pilot biscuit.

7. Add fresh or dried berries to cereal.

8. Add bran or oatmeal to ground beef.

9. Add beans, peas, or lentils to stews and chili.

10. For a low fat snack with fibre, try fig bars.

11. Eat oatmeal cookies as a sweet source of fibre.

12. Add a fresh tomato to salads or sandwiches.

13. Eat dried fruit or berries for a snack.

14. Eat the skin of fruits and potatoes.

15. Eat a fruit instead of drinking a glass of juice.

16. As a thickener, add oatmeal to duck or goose soup.

Summary of Points to Mention:

1. **To maintain a balanced diet, include a source of fibre in every meal and snack.**

Cooking with Fibre

Hearty Carrot Muffins

1 1/4 cups	whole wheat flour	300 mL
1 1/4 cups	bran cereal	300 mL
1 tsp	baking powder	5 mL
1 tsp	baking soda	5 mL
2 tsp	cinnamon	10 mL
1/2 tsp	allspice	2 mL
1/2 tsp	salt	2 mL
2	eggs	2
1 cup	grated carrots	250 mL
3/4 cup	milk	175 mL
1 tsp	vinegar	5 mL
1/3 cup	brown sugar	75 mL
1/4 cup	vegetable oil	50 mL
1/4 cup	sunflower seeds	50 mL
1/4 cup	raisins	50 mL

1. Combine flour, cereal, baking powder, baking soda, cinnamon, salt, and allspice in a large bowl. Set aside.

2. In a separate bowl, mix sugar, oil, eggs, and carrots. Combine the milk and vinegar in a measuring cup, then add to mixture.

3. Add the dry ingredients to the second bowl and mix. Add the seeds and raisins.

4. Spoon the batter into lined muffin tins. Bake for 20 minutes at 400°F (200°C). Makes 1 dozen muffins.

Adapted from: Bishop-MacDonald and Howard 1990

Grandma's Cranberry Muffins

1 cup	rolled oats	250 mL
1 1/2 cups	whole wheat flour	375 mL
1 cup	brown sugar	250 mL
2 tsp	baking powder	10 ml
1/2 tsp	salt	2 mL
1/2 tsp	cinnamon	2 mL
1/2 cup	margarine	125 mL
1 1/2 cups	chopped cranberries	375 mL
2 tsp	orange juice	10 mL
2/3 cup	milk	150 mL
1	egg	1

1. Combine oats, flour, sugar, baking powder, cinnamon and salt.

2. Blend margarine into this dry mixture until it crumbles.

3. Add cranberries.

4. Mix the orange juice, milk and egg together in a separate bowl.

5. Add the mixture of liquids to the dry mixture.

5. Spoon into lightly greased or paper lined teflon muffin tins. Bake for 20 - 25 minutes at 400°F (200°C).

Adapted from: Bishop-Macdonald and Howard 1990

Filling up on Fibre

Objective: To demonstrate how to make healthy choices that are high in fibre.

Materials: - copies of the **"Fibre Game"**
 - pencils or pens

Activity:

1. Distribute copies of the **"Fibre Game"**.

2. Read each question and the choices of answers to the group.

3. Ask participants to circle their answers on their copy of the game.

4. Draw the chart below onto a board or flip chart.

5. On the chart, record the total number of answers chosen in each category by the group. For example, if 3 of 5 people chose "B", 1 of the 5 chose "A", and 1 of the 5 chose "D" for Question #1, write those totals in the appropriate squares. Participants will then see how they scored individually, and as a group.

GroupScoring

CHOICE	#1	#2	#3	#4	#5	TOTAL
A						
B						
C						
D						

6. Read the following to the group:

- If you answered mostly a's and c's, congratulations! You are making very healthy choices. If you answered mostly b's and d's, you may want to slowly increase your dietary fibre by eating more fruit, vegetables, and whole grain breads and cereals. Discuss some foods that you think are high in fibre. (Examples: oat bran cereals, blackberries, raspberries, blueberries, whole wheat bread, Red River cereal, etc.)

Summary of Points to Mention:

1. The game provides only some examples of food choices that are high in fibre. Many of the food choices in the questions contain fibre, however only some contain large amounts.

2. It is easy to add fibre to the diet (refer to the activity **Fibre Everyday**). Increase dietary fibre slowly and drink more fluids such as water, milk, or fruit juice, to help the body handle the increased bulk created by the fibre.

3. Increasing dietary fibre helps the digestive system maintain regularity and reduces the risk of certain diseases.

The Fibre Game

The **Fibre Game** provides food options for meals or snacks. Many choices are similar in nutrient value, but differ in fibre content. Fibre is found in fruits, vegetables, whole grain breads, and cereals. Choosing foods high in fibre may be a challenge, but this game will help you become more aware of healthier choices

1. For **breakfast** you enjoy eating...

    a. oatmeal and milk
    b. coffee
    c. a bran muffin
    d. a danish

2. For **dessert** you enjoy eating ice cream. To the ice cream you add...

    a. blackberries
    b. chocolate sauce
    c. an oatmeal cookie
    d. whipped cream

3. For a **snack** you eat...

    a. cooked blueberries with a piece of bannock
    b. apple juice and a buttered pilot biscuit
    c. an apple
    d. tea and a doughnut

4. For **supper** you have roast caribou and...

    a. baked beans
    b. instant mashed potatoes
    c. baked potatoes with the skin
    d. fries and gravy

5. For a **salad in a restaurant**, you order...

    a. fresh carrots and broccoli with dip
    b. macaroni salad
    c. bean salad
    d. lettuce salad

Fibre Review

Give five good sources of dietary fibre.

1. _____

2. _____

3. _____

4. _____

5. _____

Give three reasons why dietary fibre is important.

1. _____

2. _____

3. _____

Cutting Down on Total Fat

Objective: To demonstrate how to make healthy choices involving low fat meals and snacks.

Materials:
- copies of the **"Total Fat"** quiz.
- pencils or pens

Activity:

1. Distribute a copy of the **"Total Fat"** quiz.

2. Read each question and the choice of answers to the group.

3. Encourage the group to circle their answers on their copy of the game.

4. Draw the chart below onto a board or flip chart.

5. On the chart, record the total number of answers chosen in each category by the group. For example, if 3 of 5 people chose "B", 1 of the 5 chose "A", and 1 of the 5 chose "D" for Question #1, write those totals in the appropriate squares. Participants will then see how they scored individually, and as a group.

Group Scoring

CHOICE	#1	#2	#3	#4	#5	TOTAL
A						
B						
C						
D						

6. Read the following to the group:

- If you answered mostly a's and c's, congratulations! You are making very healthy choices. If you answered mostly b's and d's, you may want to decrease total dietary fat by choosing foods that contain little or no added fat.

7. Use the **Fat Review** sheet (p. 60) and the **General Evaluation** sheet (p. 67) to evaluate what was learned.

Summary of Points to Mention:

1. Choosing foods that are low in fat may help reduce the risk of heart disease.

2. Children require many "healthy choice" foods to grow and develop properly. They need foods with high nutrient value rather than foods with high fat and/or sugar content.

3. Keep in mind that the quiz is trying to illustrate the **healthiest** choices. Although many food choices in the quiz contain valuable nutrients, some foods contain more added fat than others. An important part of healthy eating involves cutting down on total fat.

4. When choosing foods from a menu, consider how the food was prepared. Many restaurant foods are deep fried in fat and/or soaked in gravy. Choose foods that are lower in total fat, such as roasted, baked or grilled meats. Ask for salad dressing on the side, so that you can control the amount of fat on your salad.

Total Fat Quiz

The **purpose** of the **Total Fat Quiz** is to show foods that are similar in nutrient value but differ in total fat. A major difference is the extra fat added during preparation. This quiz is intended to increase your knowledge of choices that will cut down your total fat intake.

When you answer each question, consider why you chose that particular food. No answer is wrong; however, some choices may be healthier.

1. When you are at a **restaurant for supper**, you decide to order..

    a. roast beef with mixed vegetables and a baked potato
    b. french fries with gravy
    c. spaghetti in tomato sauce
    d. fried chicken nuggets and dipping sauce

2. You are not very hungry for **breakfast**, but you decide to eat...

    a. cereal with milk
    b. waffles and syrup
    c. toast with jam
    d. a doughnut

3. While you are preparing supper, you **snack** on...

    a. dried salmon
    b. chocolate bar
    c. fresh vegetables
    d. potato chips

4. For an **evening snack**, you enjoy...

    a. air popped popcorn
    b. potato chips
    c. pilot biscuit and a slice of cheese
    d. deep fried bannock

5. For **lunch** you enjoy eating....

    a. a roast moose meat sandwich and salad
    b. battered fish and chips
    c. vegetable soup with baked bannock
    d. fried moose meat and hash browns

Fat Review

1. List three ways we can cut down on the total fat we eat.

   a. _____

   b. _____

   c. _____

2. Name three pairs of similar kinds of foods, that illustrate a food that is high in fat and one that is low in fat (e.g. sour cream is high in fat, yogurt is lower in fat).

	High Fat	vs	**Lower Fat**
a.	_____		_____
b.	_____		_____
c.	_____		_____

3. Name three ways to lower the amount of fat used in food preparation.

   a. _____

   b. _____

   c. _____

4. Too much fat increases risk of what conditions?

   _____   _____   _____

Learning from Elders

Objective: To educate children about various uses of traditional foods, as described by elders in the community.

Materials: - fresh or canned fruit and/or vegetables, or a special food to give as a gift to the elder

Activity:

1. Invite an elder from the community to be a guest in your classroom.

2. Ask the elder to speak to the children about preparation and preservation methods of traditional foods, as done in the past and at present times.

3. Afterward, encourage the children to share a short story about how their parents and grandparents prepare and preserve food. Encourage the children to draw a picture of the method used to go along with the story.

Summary of points to mention:

1. Asking an elder to share stories about traditional foods may encourage young people to take pride in their traditions and to maintain these practices.

The Snacking Game

Objective: To encourage choosing healthy snacks using both traditional and market foods.

Materials: - none or food examples from below if facilities permit (suggest that each participant should bring his/her favourite snack)

Activity:

1. Encourage participants to share a favourite snack food.

2. Discuss whether the snack is a traditional or market food and to which food group(s) it belongs.

3. Discuss how to include more traditional foods as healthy snacks.

4. Distribute a copy of the list of **Healthy Snacks** provided on the next page.

5. Discuss why each food on the list is a healthy choice, and for whom it is suitable.

Summary of points to mention:

1. Choose snacks that are low in fat and high in fibre.

2. Combine foods from more than one food group (e.g., fruit and cheese.)

3. Remember that many market foods such as potato chips and pop contain a lot of fat, sugar, and/or salt, which are not healthy choices. If you choose these foods, try to limit the amount that you eat.

4. Including healthy traditional foods as part of daily snacks will provide many important nutrients.

Healthy Snacks

1. Dried caribou or moose

2. Cheese melted on baked bannock

3. Fresh berries

4. Apple juice or other fruit juice.

5. Fruit crystals enriched with vitamin C, (e.g., Tang or Quench). **Check the label for added vitamin C on other brands.** (Fruit crystals contain more sugar than natural juices, and are therefore less nutritious; however, they are also less expensive and more convenient when refrigeration is not available.)

6. Home-made milkshake with berries

7. Dried salmon

8. Cooked or dried berries

9. Oatmeal cookies

10. Fresh or dried fruit

11. Canned or dried salmon and pilot biscuits

12. Popcorn (made without oil: e.g., air popped or microwave) seasoned with your favourite spice instead of butter

13. Peanut butter sandwich

Community Action

Objective: To increase physical activity through the organization and participation in community events.

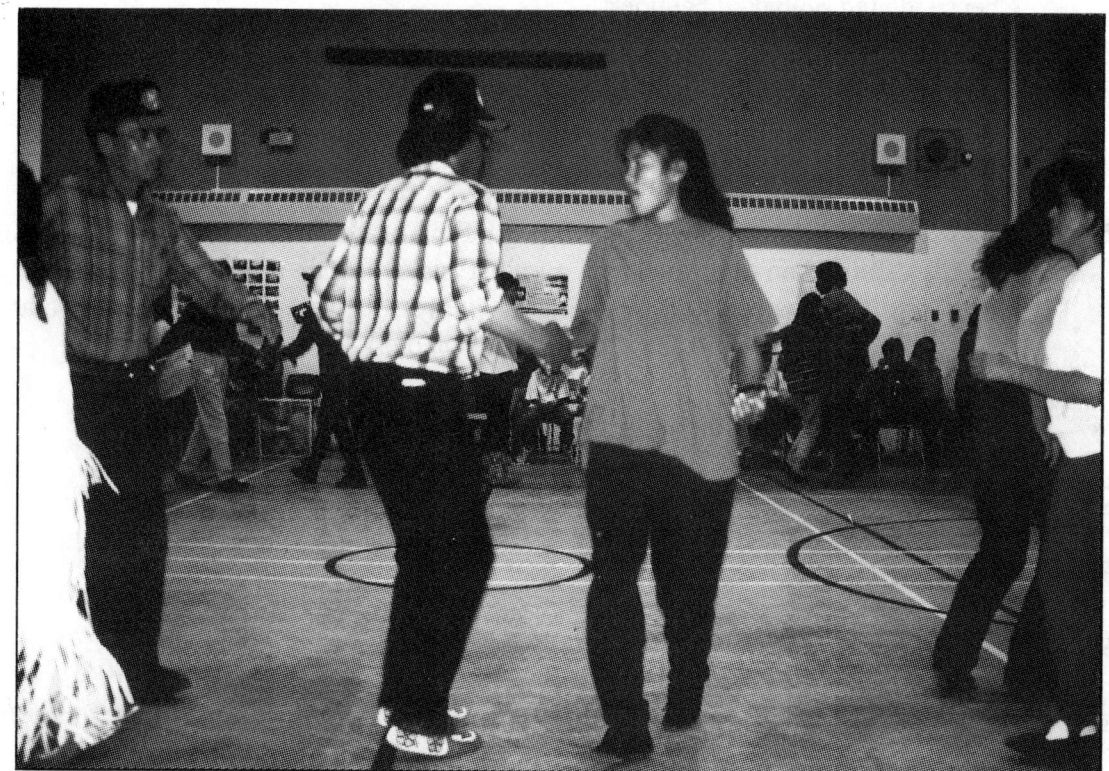

Figure 14. Dancing - a fun way to be physically active. (L to R, Steven Frost Sr., Kias Peter, and Cheryl Charlie). See activity 3 next page. (Photo: E.E. Wein)

Activity # 1: Activity Day

1. Choose a specific day to promote **Activity Day.**

2. Encourage everyone in the community to do some type of physical exercise on that particular day. This can be any type of activity, including:

   - Walking
   - Dancing
   - Swimming
   - Jigging

   - Baseball
   - Berry picking
   - Fishing
   - Sports

Activity # 2: Community Walkathon

1. Encourage other community service workers such as teachers, nurses, or social workers to advertise the **Community Walkathon**. Participants should make up and participate as teams of 2 or 3 people.

2. As a community, decide upon the distance and location/route for the walkathon. Challenge a neighbouring community to see who can attract the most participants to the event.

3. Encourage each participant to donate one can of fruit or vegetables as an entry fee. The team that finishes first will win the donated food.

Activity # 3: Community Dance-athon

1. Encourage community members of all ages to participate in a **Community Dance-athon**. Participants should have a dancing partner.

2. Reserve a community hall or school gym for the location. Encourage each couple to donate a can of fruit or vegetables as an entry fee.

3. The dance-athon should be scheduled for 12 hours with 10 minute breaks every hour and one 30 minute break after 6 hours for refreshments.

4. The team that can dance the longest without stopping, (except for the designated breaks) wins the donated food.

Activity # 4: Community Clean Up

1. Encourage young community members to donate some of their time to helping elders in the community with household activities. Many regular chores or activities would be helpful and welcomed, such as:

    - weeding the garden
    - house cleaning
    - mowing the lawn
    - baking bannock
    - preparing a meal
    - chopping firewood
    - shovelling snow
    - carrying laundry

Activity # 5: Sofa Aerobics

1. This is a great activity for those who are limited to doing minimal levels of physical activity, such as some elders. This routine will illustrate how some simple movements will help keep your muscles toned and stretched without too much exertion. It is suggested that you do each activitiy for about two minutes each, for a maximum of ten total minutes of exercise per day, to start.

2. Instructions: While you are sitting...

    a) Stretch your arms and hands as far as you can, extending the right and then the left arm, and then both arms several times.

    b) Stretch your legs and feet and keep stretching while you wiggle the toes of your right foot, and then your left foot.

    c) Move your right ankle and then your left ankle in a circular motion.

    d) Straighten and bend your right leg, and then your left leg several times.

    e) Relax, and drink some water. You have just completed **Sofa Aerobics!**

You can increase the length of time you do these exercises gradually, if desired.

General Evaluation for Games and Activities

To the educator: Use this **General Evaluation Form** as a tool to evaluate the effectiveness of the games and activities used from this handbook, and as a guide for making improvements for future use.

To the participant -

* What did you learn from this activity?

* What did you like the MOST about this activity?

* What did you like the LEAST about this activity?

* How would you improve this activity?

ADDITIONAL RESOURCES

For additional nutrition education materials, contact the organizations listed.

B.C. Heart & Stroke Foundation
1212 West Broadway
Vancouver, B.C V6H 3V2
Phone: (800) 663-2010

Health Education Associates Inc.
Pamphlet: "How to Nurse Your Baby"
8 Jan Sebastian Way
Sandwich, MA 02563
Phone: (508) 888-8044

Canadian Cancer Society
103-107 Main Street
Whitehorse, Yukon, Y1A 2A7
Phone: (867) 668-6440

First Nation Health Program Manager
Yukon Region Medical Services Branch
100 - 300 Main Street
Whitehorse, Yukon Y1A 2B5
Phone: (867) 393-6770

Dairy Nutrition Council of Alberta
14904-121A Avenue
Edmonton, Alberta, T5V 1A3
Phone: (403) 453-5942

Nutritionist
Whitehorse General Hospital
5 Hospital Road
Whitehorse, Yukon Y1A 3H7
Phone (867) 667-8700

Council for Yukon First Nations
Health and Social Development Program
Booklet: Food from the Land; Health
for the Mind, Body and Spirit.
11 Nisutlin Drive
Whitehorse, Yukon Y1A 3S4
Phone: (867) 667-7631
Fax (867) 668-6577

First Nations Health Program
Whitehorse General Hospital
5 Hospital Road
Whitehorse, Yukon Y1A 3H7
Phone (867) 667-8780

Aboriginal Diabetes Wellness Program
10959 - 102 Street
Edmonton, Albertra T5H 2V1
Phone (403) 477-4512
FAX: (403) 491-5878

REFERENCES

Bishop MacDonald, H. and Howard, M. 1990. Eat Well Live Well: The Canadian Dietetic Association's Guide to Healthy Eating, Toronto: Macmillan of Canada.

Canadian Paediatric Society, Indian and Inuit Health Committee. 1988. Vitamin D supplementation for northern native communities. Canadian Medical Association Journal 138: 229-230.

Canadian Dietetic Association. 1995. Report of the national workshop on the primary prevention of neural tube defects. Journal of the Canadian Dietetic Association 56: 167-172.

Council for Yukon Indians. c1989 Food from the Land; Health for the Mind, Body and Spirit. Whitehorse:Council for Yukon Indians.

McClellan, C. 1987. Part of the Land, Part of the Water. A History of the Yukon Indians. Vancouver: Douglas & McIntyre.

McClellan, C. 1975. My Old People Say. An Ethnographic Survey of Southern Yukon Territory. Part 1. National Museum of Man, Publications in Ethnology, No. 6(1). Ottawa: National Museums of Canada.

Medical Services Branch. 1994. Native Foods and Nutrition: An Illustrated Reference Manual. Ottawa: Health Canada.

The Ontario Milk Marketing Board. 1990. Cook Milk in Any Flavour You Like. Mississauga: Ontario Milk Marketing Board.

Walker, M. 1984. Harvesting the Northern Wild. Yellowknife: The Northern Publishers.

Wein, E.E. 1994. Yukon First Nations Food and Nutrition Study: Report to the Champagne and Aishihik First Nations, the Teslin Tlingit Council, the Vuntut Gwich'in First Nation, the Yukon Dept. of Health, and the National Institute of Nutrition. Edmonton, Alberta. Canadian Circumpolar Institute, University of Alberta. (Copies available in the named band offices, at Council for Yukon First Nations, at Yukon Health, and Yukon College Library.)

Wein, E.E. 1995. Nutrient intakes of First Nations people in four Yukon communities. Nutrition Research 15: 1105-1119.

Wein, E.E. 1996. Foods and nutrients in reported diets versus perceived ideal diets of Yukon Indian people. Journal of Nutrition Education 28: 202-208.

Wein, E. E. and Freeman, M.M.R. 1995. Frequency of traditional food use by three Yukon First Nations living in four communities. Arctic 48: 161-171.

Photos on inside back cover:

Figure 15:   Florence Smarch of Teslin with smoked whitefish. (Photo: V.M. Nardelli)
Figure 16:   Caribou meat - a source of protein, iron, zinc, and B vitamins. (Photo: E.E. Wein)
Figure 17:   The Smarch family garden in Teslin produces a variety of vegetables. (Photo: E.E. Wein)
Figure 18:   People of all ages enjoy moosemeat, as shown here by Kecia and Danny Kassi of Old Crow. (Photo: E.E. Wein)
Figure 19:   Chinook salmon eggs. (Photo: R. Chambers)
Figure 20:   Traditional and market foods served at a feast in Old Crow. (Photo: E.E. Wein)

Photos on outside back cover:

Figure 21:   Edith Josie of Old Crow cutting moose meat (Photo: E.E. Wein)
Figure 22:   Gopher (arctic ground squirrel) - a traditional Southern Tutchone food (Photo: R.W. Wein)
Figure 23:   Leafy green vegetables provide Vitamins A, C, and folate. (Photo: E.E. Wein).
Figure 24:   Fireweed shoots and leaves are a traditional source of Vitamin C. (Photo: E.E. Wein)

APPENDIX I

Canada's Food Guide to Healthy Eating

Enjoy a variety of foods from each group every day.

Choose lower-fat foods more often.

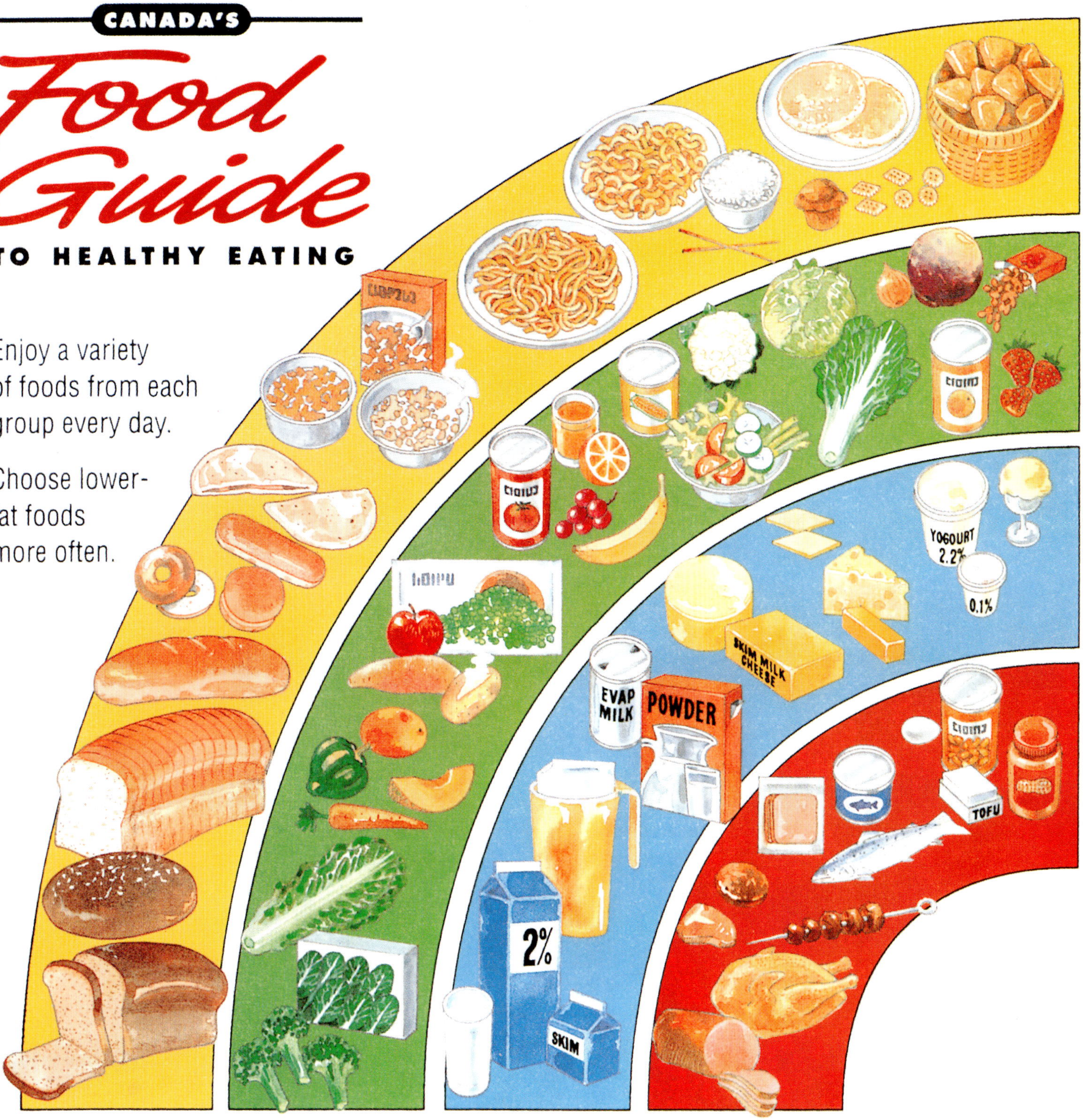

Grain Products
Choose whole grain and enriched products more often.

Vegetables & Fruit
Choose dark green and orange vegetables and orange fruit more often.

Milk Products
Choose lower-fat milk products more often.

Meat & Alternatives
Choose leaner meats, poultry and fish, as well as dried peas, beans and lentils more often.

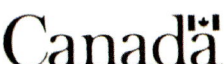

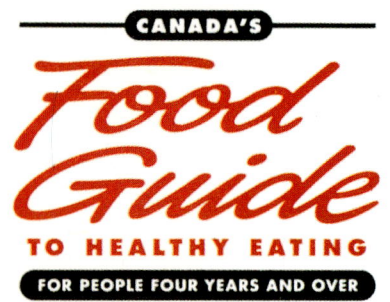

CANADA'S Food Guide TO HEALTHY EATING
FOR PEOPLE FOUR YEARS AND OVER

Different People Need Different Amounts of Food

The amount of food you need every day from the 4 food groups and other foods depends on your age, body size, activity level, whether you are male or female and if you are pregnant or breast-feeding. That's why the Food Guide gives a lower and higher number of servings for each food group. For example, young children can choose the lower number of servings, while male teenagers can go to the higher number. Most other people can choose servings somewhere in between.

Grain Products — 5–12 SERVINGS PER DAY

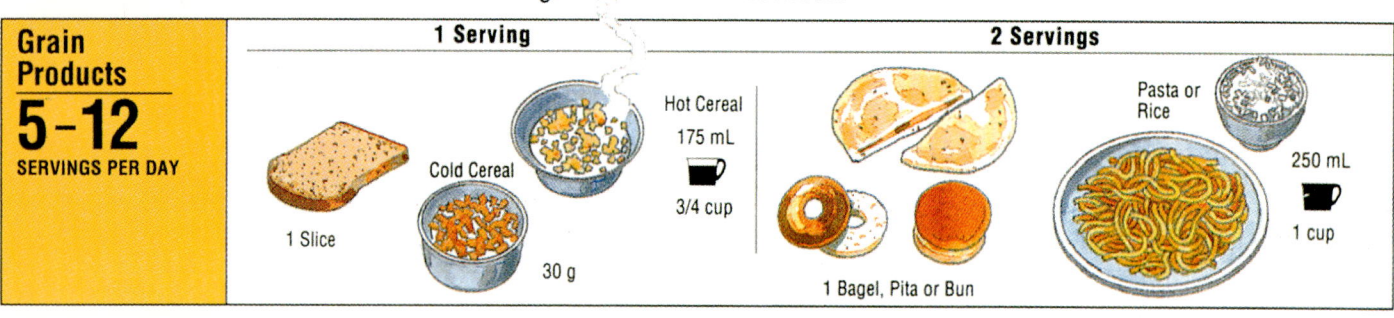

Vegetables & Fruit — 5–10 SERVINGS PER DAY

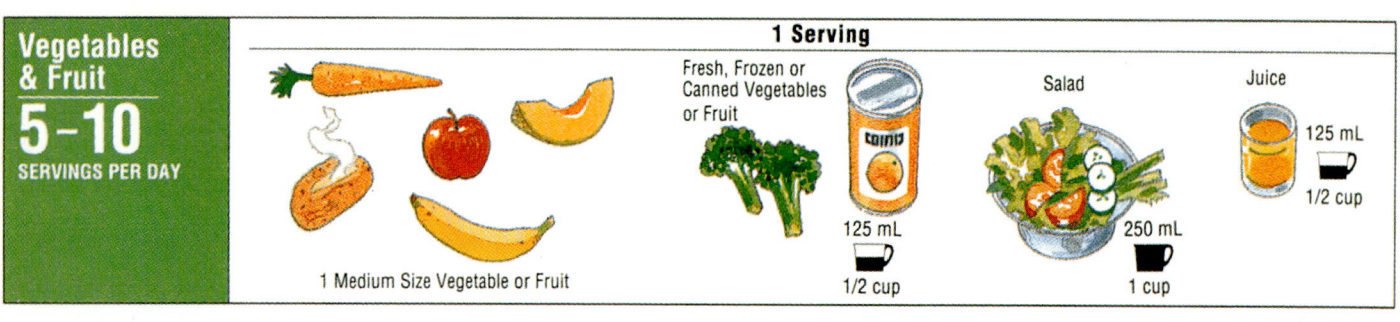

Milk Products — SERVINGS PER DAY
Children 4–9 years: 2–3
Youth 10–16 years: 3–4
Adults: 2–4
Pregnant & Breast-feeding Women: 3–4

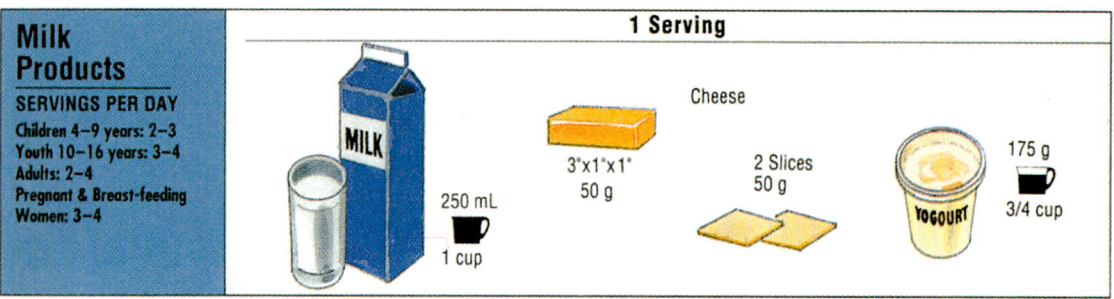

Other Foods

Taste and enjoyment can also come from other foods and beverages that are not part of the 4 food groups. Some of these foods are higher in fat or Calories, so use these foods in moderation.

Meat & Alternatives — 2–3 SERVINGS PER DAY

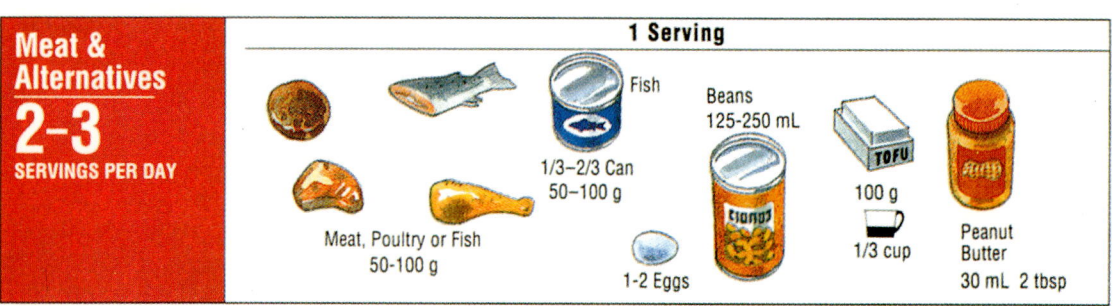

Enjoy eating well, being active and feeling good about yourself. That's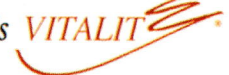

© Minister of Supply and Services Canada 1992   Cat. No. H39-252/1992E   No changes permitted. Reprint permission not required.
ISBN 0-662-19648-1